Point-of-Care Ultrasound Fundamentals: Principles, Devices, and Patient Safety

Point-of-Care Ultrasound Fundamentals: Principles, Devices, and Patient Safety

Paul R. Wagner, BS, RDMS, RDCS, RVT
Program Director
Diagnostic Medical Sonography
South Hills School of Business and Technology
State College, Pennsylvania

Wayne R. Hedrick, PhD, FACR
Northeast Ohio Medical University
Rootstown, Ohio
Aultman Hospital
Canton, Ohio

Mc Graw Hill Education | Medical

New York   Chicago   San Francisco   Athens   London   Madrid   Mexico City
Milan   New Delhi   Singapore   Sydney   Toronto

Point-of-Care Ultrasound Fundamentals: Principles, Devices, and Patient Safety

ISBN 978-0-07-183002-7
MHID 0-07-183002-2

This book was set in BerkeleyStd-Book by MPS Limited.
The editors were Andrew Moyer and Regina Y. Brown.
The production supervisor was Catherine H. Saggese.
Production management was provided by Charu Khanna at MPS Limited.
China Translation & Printing Services, Ltd. was printer and binder.

This book is printed on acid-free paper.

Library of Congress Cataloging-in-Publication Data

Wagner, Paul R. (Sonography educator), author.
  Point-of-Care Ultrasound Fundamentals: Principles, Devices, and Patient Safety / Paul R. Wagner and Wayne R. Hedrick. —
First edition.
     p. ; cm.
  Includes bibliographical references and index.
  ISBN 978-0-07-183002-7 (pbk. : alk. paper) — ISBN 0-07-183002-2 (pbk. : alk. paper)
  I. Hedrick, Wayne R., author. II. Title.
  [DNLM: 1. Ultrasonography—methods. 2. Patient Safety. 3. Point-of-Care Systems. WN 208]
  RC78.7.U4
  616.07'543—dc23
                                                            2014007929

McGraw-Hill books are available at special quantity discounts to use as premiums and sales promotions, or for use in corporate training programs. To contact a representative please visit the Contact Us pages at www.mhprofessional.com.

To Fred Thompson: Engineer, entrepreneur, barbershopper, friend
(PRW)

To Drs. James and Esther Rehmus: To curiosity and adventure.
(WRH)

Contents

Preface

Since the mid-1970s, the medical imaging community has been transmitting sound energy into the human body, noninvasively, to obtain diagnostic information. In the intervening 40 years, sonography has expanded in complexity and application to become an invaluable tool in the diagnostic arsenal of almost every traditional medical specialty.

Diagnostic ultrasonography has revolutionized the prenatal diagnosis of abnormalities of the fetus and has further expanded to diagnose diseases in the abdomen, pelvis, thyroid, prostate, breast, heart, blood vessels, and neonatal brain. In many cases, the development of new sonographic techniques has supplanted previous, antiquated diagnostic methods. A good example of this is the venous duplex examination that has completely replaced other invasive and noninvasive procedures in the assessment of deep vein thrombosis.

Recently, the use of ultrasound in "nontraditional" and primary care environments has grown exponentially. With the advantages of relatively low cost, portability, and wide range of applications, sonography has become a first-line diagnostic tool in developing countries. Medical education has adopted ultrasonography as a part of the core medical school curriculum, and the modality is now being referred to as the stethoscope of the future. These factors combine to increase clinical utilization and to make worldwide ultrasound equipment sales higher in revenue than all other imaging modalities, including magnetic resonance imaging and computed tomography.

Many "new" ultrasound practitioners do not have traditional medical imaging training and, therefore, they have not been exposed to the foundational principles of medical ultrasound physics. Ultrasound is often considered completely harmless by the community at large and, thus, is presumed it can be used without constraint as one would pick up a flashlight to investigate a darkened corner.

Although a myriad of scientific studies conducted in parallel with growth of the modality reinforce the belief that ultrasound is relatively safe, several important points must be stressed.

First, a sound wave is the mechanical vibrations of molecules within a medium. At power levels achievable with currently available diagnostic equipment, high frequency sound energy has the potential to increase temperature of the tissue and damage cells, particularly when scanning the fetus. To avoid harm, operators must have a basic understanding of ultrasound interactions with tissue as well as the equipment controls and display parameters that affect the amount of energy transmitted into the patient.

Second, any exposure of the human body to ultrasound energy must be viewed from the perspective of risk versus benefit. The benefit may be medical or educational. Even when the risk is very small, the risk always outweighs the benefit when no medical or educational benefit can be demonstrated. The practice of diagnostic ultrasound should always incorporate the ALARA principle, "As Low As Reasonably Achievable." ALARA applies to equipment parameters and application presets, examination time, observance of Output Display Indices, and training (including credentialing when available) of the operator.

Finally, a study in 2009 showed that a very high percentage of ultrasound professionals are working in pain, largely due to improper body positioning and scanning technique. Proper positioning and scanning techniques are essential in obtaining the optimal diagnostic images as well as avoiding musculoskeletal injuries to the ultrasound practitioner.

This book is a powerful tool that can provide a basic understanding of the physics of sound interactions with tissue and the equipment controls that allow the user to maximize the quality of diagnostic information obtained during the ultrasound examination. Universal scanning techniques are described in detail (Chapter 9), with diagrams and photographs used to illustrate correct (and incorrect) scanning techniques. These techniques are applicable to every type of ultrasound procedure, and begin at the most basic level by addressing the proper transducer grip.

The need for the point-of-care ultrasound community to have a resource that explains the fundamentals of diagnostic ultrasound has long been recognized. We hope this book explains these principles clearly in an easy to understand format.

Paul R. Wagner, BS, RDMS, RDCS, RVT
Wayne R. Hedrick, PhD, FACR

Acknowledgments

The authors would like to thank the following individuals for their help in obtaining images and photographs for this text:

Elizabeth Ladrido BS, RDMS, RVT
Linda Metzger, RT, RDMS, RVT
Gregory Tressler, RT(R), RDMS
Tricia Turner, BS, RDMS, RVT
McKenzee Walker, AST

We would also like to thank the following manufacturers for their support of this project:

FUJIFILM-Sonosite, Inc
GE Healthcare
Philips Healthcare
Sound Ergonomics, LLC

Basic Ultrasound Physics

OBJECTIVES

- To define common descriptors of ultrasound waves.
- To state the relationship between acoustic velocity, wavelength, and frequency.
- To describe the types of ultrasound interactions with tissue.

- To recognize the importance of the acoustic impedance mismatch at the interface in specular reflection.
- To understand the frequency dependence of attenuation in tissue.
- To explain the principle of echo ranging.

KEY TERMS

Absorption
Acoustic impedance
Acoustic velocity
Attenuation
Compression
Echo ranging
Frequency
Intensity
Interference
Longitudinal wave

Power
Propagation
Rarefaction
Reflectivity
Refraction
Scattering
Specular reflection
Transducer
Wavelength

SOUND

Sound is mechanical energy that is transmitted through a medium (e.g., air, water, metal, or tissue) by forces acting on molecules. The induced molecular motion is periodic whereby the molecules oscillate back and forth about their unperturbed positions. These fluctuations cause variations in molecular density and pressure (greater than and lower than the natural state) along the path of the sound wave. As vibrating molecules (also referred to as particles) interact with their neighbors, the periodic changes in pressure and molecular density are conveyed from one location to another. The term propagation describes this transmittal of mechanical energy to distant regions remote from the sound source.

Compression and Rarefaction

Consider the motion of the diaphragm in an audio speaker as a sound source. When the diaphragm moves forward, the air molecules immediately in front are pushed together, producing a region of increased air density, and correspondingly increased pressure. The term compression describes the formation of the high-pressure region (Figure 1-1). When the diaphragm reverses direction, a zone of decreased air density results. The term rarefaction describes the creation of this low-pressure region.

The vibration of the diaphragm alternately compresses the air on a forward thrust and rarefies the air on a backward thrust. The regions of compression and rarefaction are transmitted through the medium by molecular interactions. The originally affected molecules collide with adjacent molecules to propagate the action of the diaphragm. Thus, the transmission of mechanical energy through the medium creates regions of varying particle density and pressure. Compression zones alternate with rarefaction zones. Between adjacent compression zones, particle density decreases from a maximum in the compression zone to a minimum in the rarefaction zone and then increases back to a maximum at the succeeding compression zone.

If the action of sound propagation is frozen in time, a plot of particle density as a function of distance exhibits a sinusoidal wave pattern (Figure 1-2A). At a later instant in time, the sinusoidal wave pattern of particle density is maintained (Figure 1-2B), but the compression and rarefaction zones have shifted to new locations along the direction of propagation. This is described as linear propagation since molecular density follows a sine wave variation along the

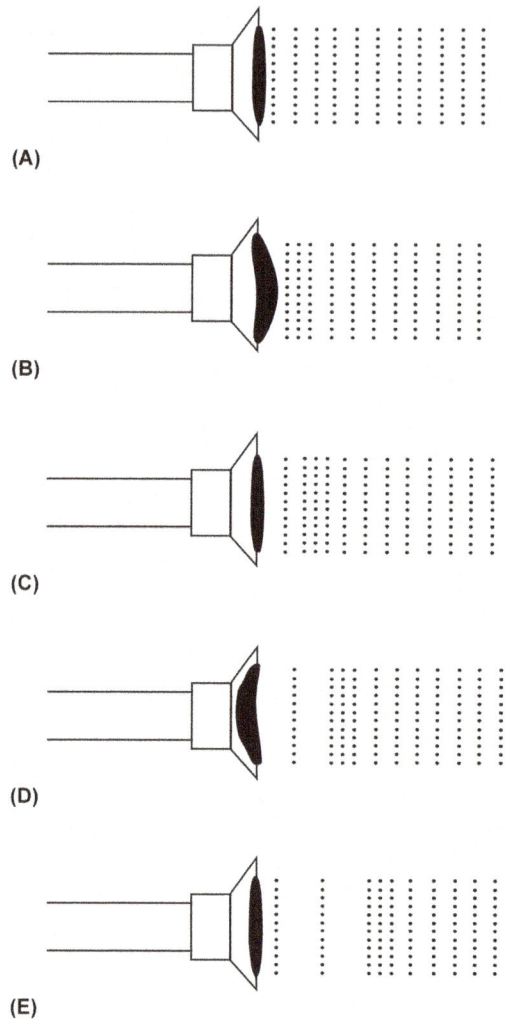

(A)

(B)

(C)

(D)

(E)

FIGURE 1-1. Action of the speaker alters the density of air molecules. (**A**) Undisturbed medium (no movement of diaphragm). (**B**) High-density region created by outward movement of diaphragm. (**C**) Diaphragm returning to its original position as a region of compression advances. (**D**) Low-density region created by inward movement of diaphragm. (**E**) Diaphragm returning to its original position as the regions of compression and rarefaction advance.

transmission path (plot of molecular density with distance at an instant in time is a sine wave). Molecular density is not constant at a particular location in the medium but oscillates with a certain time dependence imposed by the action of the sound source. The rate of change from high density to low density depends

(A)

(B)

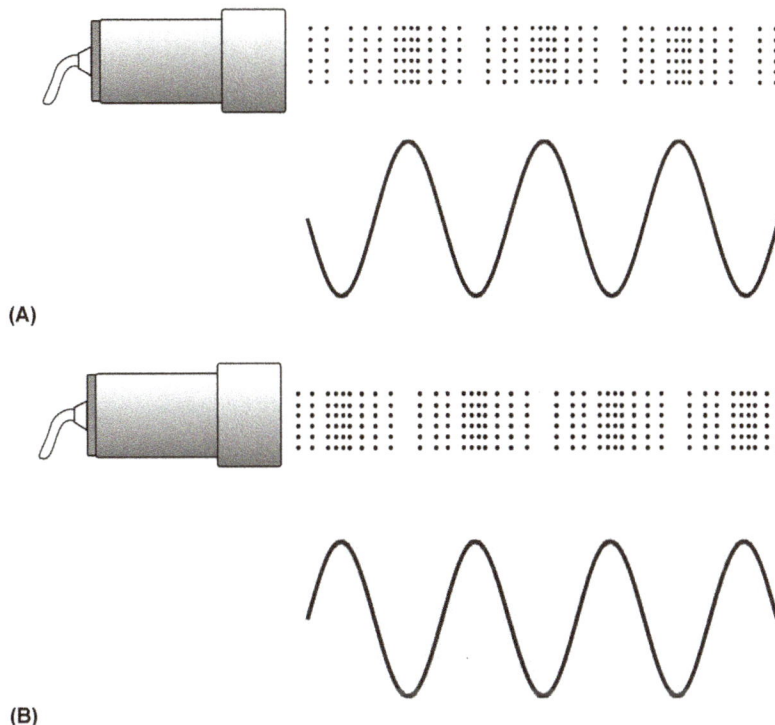

FIGURE 1-2. Particle density along the path of propagation varies with distance from the source and time. Regions of high- and low-density alternate and are transitioned by immediate density as shown by the sinusoidal curve. (**A**) At one instance in time. (**B**) A short time later the density regions are displaced to the right along the direction of propagation.

on how fast the sound source vibrates (how rapidly the diaphragm moves in and out).

The molecules are displaced from and vibrate about their customary positions (a distance of only several microns) as the sound wave passes through the medium. The motion of the molecules at a particular location is also sinusoidal and is dictated by the vibrational rate of the sound source. Molecules do not travel from one end of the medium to the other; there is no flow of particles. Rather, the effect is transmitted over long distances because of neighbor-to-neighbor interactions. Sound transmission cannot occur in a vacuum because no molecules are available to transfer the mechanical vibrations.

Sound transmission is usually portrayed diagrammatically by showing the compression zones. A compression zone is often considered the leading portion of the sound wave and hence is called the

wavefront. Wavefronts are helpful in illustrating the direction sound travels (perpendicular to the compression zone) and the region over which sound transmission takes place (the ultrasonic field).

Wave Descriptors

Amplitude is the magnitude of a physical entity from the neutral value to the maximum extent in an oscillation. The term can be applied to acoustic pressure, particle density, particle displacement, or particle velocity in the medium. It has other applications, such as to characterize the magnitude of a voltage pulse delivered to or induced within the crystal of the transducer. Since the motion of the molecules is repetitive, the term *cycle* is used to describe any sequence of changes in molecular motion (particle displacement, density of molecules, pressure, or particle velocity) that recurs at regular intervals.

The frequency of a wave is the number of vibrations (back and forth movements) that a molecule makes per second or the number of times the cycle is repeated each second. For comparative purposes, higher frequency means that the cyclic motion is executed at a faster rate and more cycles are completed in the 1-s interval than at lower frequency. Sound waves are those pressure changes that the human ear can detect. They oscillate at frequencies of 20–20,000 cycles per second or hertz (Hz). Cycle is not a standard unit of measurement but is used as a descriptor to clarify the concept of frequency. Often, frequency is expressed in units of inverse time only (1/s or s^{-1}). Ultrasound is defined as mechanical waves with higher frequency than humans can hear, frequencies greater than 20,000 Hz or 20 kHz. The frequency range for diagnostic medical ultrasound is 2–22 megahertz (MHz). Infrasound refers to mechanical waves with frequencies lower than humans can hear, frequencies less than 20 Hz. Sound and ultrasound have similar properties, and thus are often used interchangeably in the description of physical interactions.

Longitudinal waves are those in which particle motion is along the direction of the wave energy propagation; that is, the molecules vibrate back and forth in the same direction as the wave travel. Sound waves in liquids and soft tissue are longitudinal. For transverse waves, which occur in bone and metal, the particle motion is perpendicular to the direction of propagation.

Wavelength is the distance for one complete wave cycle as illustrated by the variation in particle density along the propagation path (Figure 1-3). Wavelength is measured between two successive equivalent density zones (i.e., two compression zones or two rarefaction zones) and is expressed in units of a meter (m), centimeter (cm), or millimeter (mm). The wavelength in diagnostic sonography is less than 1 mm.

The frequency of a wave is the number of cycles (pressure oscillations) occurring at a given point in 1 s. When the particle density at a point is plotted as a function of time, the period of the wave is defined as the time necessary for one complete cycle or the time between two successive compression zones or rarefaction zones. The period is equal to the

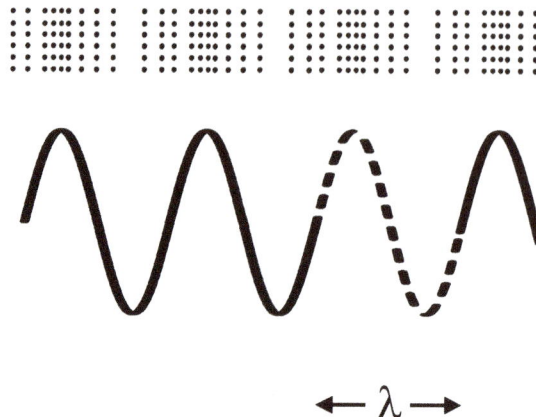

FIGURE 1-3. Particle density along the path of propagation at one instance in time. The wavelength is equal to the distance between successive maxima or minima and is defined as the distance needed to complete one wave cycle (dotted line).

reciprocal of the frequency. For example, when the frequency is halved (from 4 to 2 MHz), the period is doubled (from 2.5×10^{-7} to 5.0×10^{-7} s).

The speed at which a wave propagates through the medium (rate of transfer of the mechanical vibrations) is called the acoustic velocity. The velocity of sound depends on the physical density (mass per unit volume) and compressibility of the medium. In soft tissue, the acoustic velocity is an average of 1540 m/s. Note that the acoustic velocity is not the same as the particle velocity, which refers to the speed of the individual molecules when mechanical force is applied.

The rate at which the wave transmits energy over a small area is the intensity (expressed in units of watts per centimeter squared (W/cm^2) or milliwatts per centimeter squared (mW/cm^2)). As sound intensity is increased, the molecular density and acoustic pressure in the compression zone are also increased, which is accompanied by longer particle oscillation length and faster particle velocity. Intensity does not affect frequency, wavelength, and acoustic velocity during linear propagation. In a stereo system, the volume control adjusts the loudness of the sound output but does not alter the pitch (frequency). As volume is increased, the diaphragm moves over a greater distance, but the time for an in and out oscillation is unchanged. Power is a measure of the rate at which energy is transmitted into the medium by the transducer. Summing the intensity over the entire cross-sectional area of the ultrasonic field yields the power (expressed in watts, milliwatts, or joules per second).

SOUND-PROPAGATION MEDIA

Sound waves are mechanical in nature and they require an elastic deformable medium for propagation, which can be gas, liquid, or solid. A solid is deformable because pressure, when applied, causes a change in shape. Elasticity is demonstrated by a return to the original shape following removal of the pressure. The amount of distortion depends on the strength of the force and the elastic properties of the medium. The latter is determined by molecular interactions. Propagation of an ultrasound wave through soft tissue causes elastic deformations by the separation and grouping of neighboring molecules.

If all other physical properties of the medium are maintained unchanged, then an increase in density impedes the rate of sound propagation through the medium. As the density increases, more mass is contained within a given volume. For particles with increasingly larger mass, more force is required to produce molecular motion; and once the molecules are moving, more force is required to stop them. This is true for the rhythmic starting and stopping required to produce sound transmission. Thus, on the basis of density alone, sound is expected to have a greater velocity in air (low density) than in bone (high density). However, this is not the case and an additional factor must influence acoustic velocity.

The other physical property of a medium that affects the acoustic velocity is compressibility, the fractional decrease in volume when pressure is applied to the material. A high value for compressibility indicates that the medium is easily reduced in volume. The parameter relating the elastic properties of a medium to the acoustic velocity is usually the reciprocal of the compressibility, or the bulk modulus. Large values for the bulk modulus indicate that a material is resistant

to change in its volume when force is applied (low compressibility). Acoustic velocity is directly proportional to the square root of the bulk modulus.

A dense material (e.g., bone or other solid) is very difficult to reduce in volume when pressure is applied to it. This low compressibility predicts the high velocity of sound in bone. By contrast, air is easily reduced in volume because the gas molecules are far apart and can be easily brought closer together (compressibility is high). The velocity of sound in air is low. Based on *both* density and compressibility differences, the velocity of sound in bone (4080 m/s) is much greater than that in air (330 m/s). For liquids in general, the interdependence of density and compressibility counteract each other and consequently different liquids tend to transmit ultrasound at nearly the same velocity. In the transmission of sound, soft tissue behaves similarly to liquid; the acoustic velocities for various tissue types do not vary by more than a few percent. The average velocity of ultrasound in tissue is 1540 m/s or 154,000 cm/s or 1.54 mm/μs. Acoustic velocities for common materials are shown in Table 1-1. Generally, more dense media (most solids) have greater velocities than do less dense media (liquids or gases), because their compressibility is low.

TABLE 1-1 • Acoustic Velocity in Different Tissue

Material	Acoustic Velocity (m/s)
Liver	1555
Lung	600
Muscle	1600
Bone	4080
Fat	1460
Blood	1560
Soft tissue (average)	1540

RELATIONSHIP BETWEEN ACOUSTIC VELOCITY, WAVELENGTH, AND FREQUENCY

The acoustic velocity (c) equals the product of the frequency (f) and the wavelength (λ):

$$c = f \lambda \qquad 1\text{-}1$$

Because the acoustic velocity is constant for a particular medium, an increase in frequency causes the wavelength to decrease. The wavelength in tissue for a 2.5-MHz frequency wave is 0.62 mm. If the frequency is raised to 5 MHz, the resulting wavelength is 0.31 mm or one-half the value of 0.62 mm at 2.5 MHz, because the frequency has doubled.

When transmitted across media with different acoustic velocities, the frequency of the sound remains constant. Consequently, a change in the wavelength must accompany the velocity shift when the sound wave is propagated through different media. For the 2.5-MHz sound wave transmitted from soft tissue into bone, the wavelength increases from 0.62 to 1.6 mm.

The wavelength of the ultrasound wave as a function of frequency can be determined for any medium for which the acoustic velocity is known. In diagnostic medical sonography, the medium of interest is soft tissue where an acoustic velocity of 1540 m/s is assumed. For soft tissue, the calculation for wavelength can be simplified by dividing 1.54 by the frequency expressed in megahertz to yield the wavelength in millimeters. Table 1-2 lists the wavelength of an ultrasound wave in soft tissue as the frequency is varied.

SOUND TRANSMISSION

The sonographic image, unlike that in radiography, is typically based on reflected rather than transmitted energy. The single device that generates the ultrasound wave and, subsequently, detects the reflected echo is the transducer. The transducer may oper-

TABLE 1-2 • Frequency Dependence of Wavelength for Ultrasound in Soft Tissue	
Frequency (MHz)	Wavelength (mm)
2.5	0.62
5.0	0.31
10	0.15
15	0.10
20	0.08

ate in continuous or pulsed mode depending on the application. A continuous-wave (CW) transducer continuously emits a sound wave with constant frequency with constant peak-pressure amplitude (Figure 1-4). Pulsed-wave (PW) transmission is a short-duration burst of sound (a few cycles in length) emitted from the sound source (Figure 1-5). In the latter case, the transducer must be turned on and off very rapidly (sound generation is less than 1 μs).

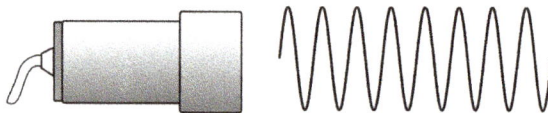

FIGURE 1-4. Continuous-wave output generated by the transducer.

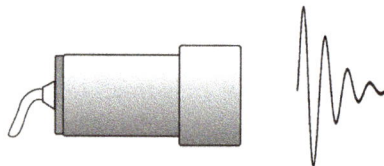

FIGURE 1-5. Pulsed-wave output generated by the transducer.

TYPES OF INTERACTIONS

The types of interactions that occur in tissue are similar to the wave behavior observed with light: reflection, refraction, scattering, divergence, interference, and absorption. The outcome of these interactions is detected in the form of reflected ultrasound waves (echoes). The overall reduction in the intensity by reflection, scattering, and absorption is called attenuation.

Specular Reflection

A major interaction of interest for diagnostic sonography is specular reflection. If a sound beam is incident on a smooth interface (e.g., the boundary between different tissue types) much larger than the wavelength of the wave, some energy is partially reflected back toward the sound source (Figure 1-6). This interaction is responsible for the major organ outlines seen in diagnostic sonography. The skull, diaphragm, and pericardium are also examples of specular reflectors. The sonogram of the fetal head in Figure 1-7 illustrates the strong echoes obtained from the skull.

At other than normal incidence, the angle of reflection of a sound beam is equal to the angle of incidence. To obtain maximum detection of the reflected echo, the transducer (which sends and receives) must be oriented so the generated sound beam strikes the interface with near perpendicularity and the reflected wave travels along a similar path back to transducer.

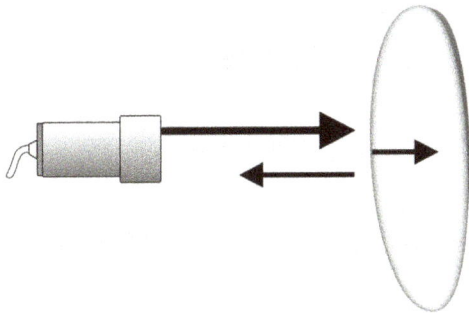

FIGURE 1-6. Reflection caused by a sound wave striking a specular reflector. The composition of the interface determines the relative intensities of the transmitted and reflected waves.

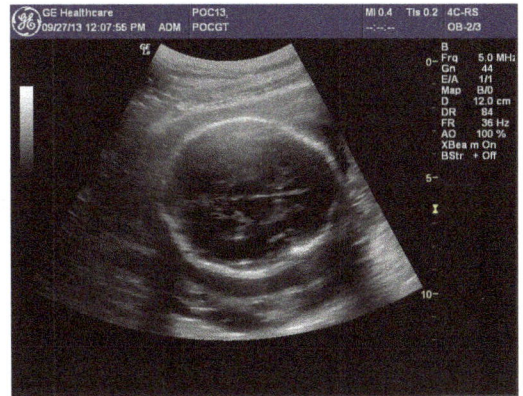

FIGURE 1-7. Sonogram of the fetal head showing strong specular reflection from the skull.

What conditions result in a reflection of energy? A useful analogy would be throwing a baseball against a brick wall; not much energy will be transferred to the wall. Conservation of energy would permit the ball to transfer all its energy to the wall and simply stop at the surface of the wall, but conservation of momentum prevents this from occurring because of the differences in mass. Only a small portion of the energy is transferred to the wall. Most is retained by the baseball, which returns with almost the same velocity as when it struck the wall.

Similarly, if a Mack truck rams into a Volkswagen, very little energy will be transferred to the Volkswagen. The truck will continue at almost the same velocity as it originally had. Most of its energy will be retained, although a great deal of damage will be done to the Volkswagen. Energy cannot be transmitted readily from large objects to small ones or from small objects to large ones. If massive transfers of kinetic energy are required, collisions between objects of equal mass must occur. For example, to slow down a baseball, the maximum amount of energy transfer will result if it collides with another baseball. To transfer energy from a Mack truck by the maximum amount, it would have to collide with another Mack truck. Vibrating molecules behave in a similar manner. As long as they are transmitting energy to identically sized molecules, maximum transfer will occur. If there is a difference in the masses of the molecules, less energy will be transferred and the energy that is not transferred will be reflected.

Acoustic Impedance

The product of density and acoustic velocity yields the acoustic impedance, which is a measure of the resistance to sound passing through the medium. Acoustic impedance is expressed in units of the rayl. High-density materials generally give rise to high-velocity sound waves and therefore high acoustic impedances. Similarly, low-density materials such as gases have low acoustic impedances. Table 1-3 lists the acoustic impedances for several materials of interest.

Impedance Mismatch

When a diver enters a pool, the ripple pattern expands outward and is reflected from the concrete wall of the pool. Very little wave energy is transferred from the water to the concrete wall. Now consider what would happen if the walls were made of Jell-O instead of concrete. The reflected wave in the water would be less intense and the walls would vibrate. Energy is transferred from the water to the Jell-O because the composition and the acoustic impedance of the two materials are similar.

If the acoustic impedance is the same in one medium as in another, sound is readily transmitted from one to the other. A difference in acoustic impedances causes some portion of the sound to be reflected at the interface. It is primarily the change in acoustic impedance at a biological interface (an impedance mismatch) that allows visualization of soft tissue structures with an ultrasonic beam. Watching late-night western movies teaches that one does not listen for the train or for buffalo in a normal standing position. Every youngster learned from old westerns that you put your ear to the rail or to the ground. The late John Wayne

TABLE 1-3 • Properties of Different Media

Material	Density (kg/m^3)	Velocity (m/s)	Acoustic Impedance (megarayls)
Air	1.2	330	0.0004
Water (20°C)	1000	1480	1.48
Soft tissue average	1060	1540	1.63
Liver	1060	1550	1.64
Muscle	1080	1580	1.7
Fat	952	1460	1.38
Kidney	1038	1560	1.62
Blood	1057	1575	1.62
Bone	1912	4080	7.8
Lung	400	600	0.24
PZT	7650	3791	29

PZT, Lead zirconate titanate.

most likely would not have said, "Put your ear to the ground because that way you will eliminate the acoustic impedance mismatch and thus get a better sound transfer," but he should have, for that is the case. Whereas the transfer of sound from rail to air and then from air to ear is very inefficient, with direct contact the transmission from rail to air is eliminated and vibrations pass readily across a solid-solid interface.

Another analogy that might be used is the transmission of light. Light transmitted from one medium to another having different indices of refraction causes the major portion of the energy to be reflected rather than transmitted. This phenomenon can be observed when looking at sunlight reflected from a shallow pool of water. The reflection occurs at the air-water boundary because of the different indices of refraction (similar to acoustic impedance). The amount of reflection is a function of the surface only. One receives the same amount of reflected light standing over a pool of water as over the deepest part of the Pacific Ocean. Sound is reflected at the interface regardless of the thickness of the material from which it is reflected.

Reflection Coefficient

For perpendicular incidence, the reflection coefficient for intensity, which equals the ratio of the reflected intensity (I_r) to the incident intensity (I_i), is proportional to the square of the difference in acoustic impedances of the media and is given by

$$\alpha_R = \frac{I_r}{I_i} = \left(\frac{Z_2 - Z_1}{Z_2 + Z_1}\right)^2 \qquad 1\text{-}2$$

where α_R is the reflection coefficient, Z_2 the acoustic impedance of medium number 2 (distal to the boundary), and Z_1 the acoustic impedance of medium number 1 (proximal to the boundary). If the reflection coefficient is known, then the transmission coefficient can be determined by subtracting the reflection coefficient from unity.

For specular reflection, transmission and reflection of energy are independent of frequency. That is, frequency does not affect the fraction of intensity transmitted and reflected at the interface.

Interface Composition

The order of the acoustic impedance for two materials that compose the interface has no effect on the reflected intensity—the difference between them squared gives the same number. *Thus, the same percentage of reflection occurs at the interface, whether sound is going from high acoustic impedance to low acoustic impedance, or vice versa.* If the acoustic impedance difference is small, the magnitude of the reflected wave is small. Because the same device transmits and receives the sound waves, maximum intensity of the detected echo occurs when the sound beam strikes the interface with near normal incidence. If the acoustic impedance difference is large, such as in bone compared to soft tissue, a large fraction of sound is reflected and the transmitted beam weakly penetrates structures behind the bone. This is one of the reasons why bone is usually avoided during an ultrasound examination. To visualize the liver, which is largely positioned under the ribs, one must direct the ultrasound beam either through the intercostal spaces (between the ribs) or under the ribs and back up at the liver.

Table 1-4 lists the fraction of the incident intensity reflected at interfaces of varying composition. The acoustic impedances obtained from Table 1-3 are used to calculate these values. Note that the thickness of the medium and frequency are not considered in the calculations; only the impedance mismatch at the interface is of concern.

The acoustic impedance difference is also large for an air-tissue interface, which causes most of the

TABLE 1-4 • Reflection at Different Interfaces

Interface	Percent Reflected
Soft tissue-air	99.9
Soft tissue-bone	43
Fat-liver	1

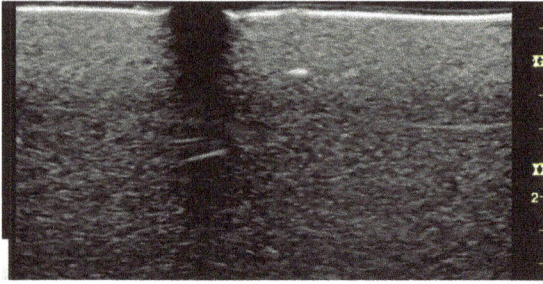

FIGURE 1-8. Example of air as a near total reflector. Sonogram of a tissue-mimicking phantom with an air bubble present between the transducer and the phantom surface. The transmission of ultrasound energy into the phantom is prevented by air creating a signal void distal to the air bubble.

incident beam to be reflected. Even if the air layer between a transducer and the patient is extremely thin, nearly total reflection occurs at the air-tissue interface. The ultrasound beam is not transmitted to structures distal to the air bubble and the sonogram is void of information from this region (Figure 1-8). During scanning, the application of coupling gel eliminates air gaps. The gel also serves to reduce friction between the transducer and the skin.

When the heart or other thoracic structures are being studied, the lungs must be avoided because of the large amount of reflection that occurs at the multiple air interfaces within them. Acoustic impedance differences at fat-soft tissue interfaces produce relatively strong echoes (~1% of the incident intensity) and are primarily responsible for the organ outlines seen in imaging.

Diffuse Reflection

The large smooth surface of a specular reflector acts as a mirror to form a well-defined, redirected beam (echo). A large rough-surfaced interface deflects the ultrasound beam in multiple directions. Since the interface is not entirely flat, the sound beam strikes the interface with various angles of incidence, which gives rise to differing angles of reflection. This is called diffuse reflection. The loss of coherence in the reflected beam weakens the echo returning to the transducer. Diffuse reflection is relatively independent of the orientation of the interface.

Before the bathroom mirror becomes fogged when you take a shower, it provides a true representation of objects placed in front of it. After you shower, the buildup of water on its surface causes it to act as a diffuse reflector and the images of objects are less well defined. Water particles roughen the mirror's surface, reducing the coherence of reflected light.

Scattering

Another extremely important interaction between ultrasound and tissue is scattering, or nonspecular reflection, which is responsible for providing the internal texture of organs in the image. The scattering occurs because the interfaces are small, with physical dimensions less than a wavelength. Each interface acts as a new separate sound source, and sound is reflected in all directions independent of the direction of the incoming sound wave (Figure 1-9). The magnitude of scattered ultrasound intensity is much weaker than for specular reflection and depends on the number of scatterers per volume, size of the scatterers, acoustic impedance, and the frequency.

Fluid regions such as cysts, urine in the bladder, and amniotic fluid lack scattering centers and produce weak ultrasound signals compared with surrounding tissue (dark areas in the image which are described as hypoechoic). Areas with increased ultrasound signals compared with the surrounding tissue are called hyperechoic. The sonogram of the fetus in Figure 1-10 illustrates low and high signal variations throughout the scanned tissues.

Scattering by extremely small particles in which the dimensions are very much less than the

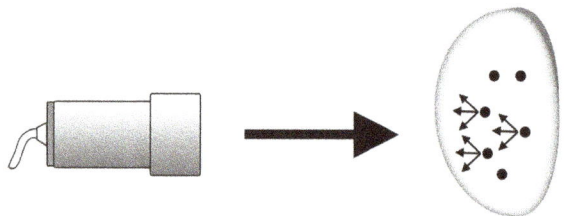

FIGURE 1-9. Scattering. Small structures redirect the sound energy in all directions. The direction of the scattered waves is relatively independent of the incident beam direction.

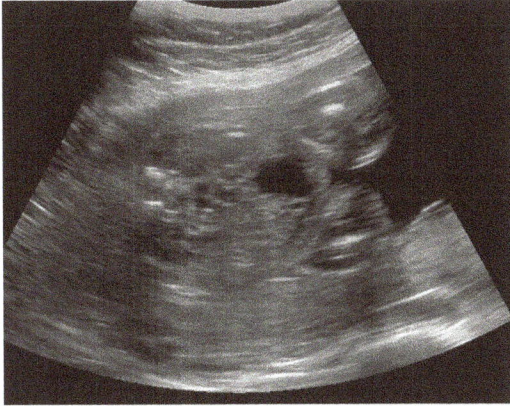

FIGURE 1-10. Cross-sectional image of a fetal abdomen. Amniotic fluid (dark area to the right on the image) is relatively echo free (hypoechoic), while bone (brightest white areas in the image) produces high signal levels (hyperechoic). Soft tissue has intermediate signal levels. The circular hypoechoic structure near the middle of the image is the fetal urinary bladder.

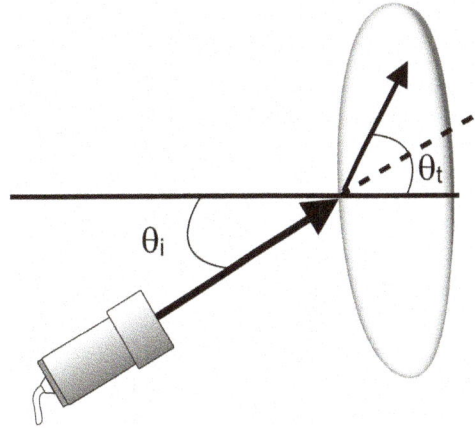

FIGURE 1-11. Refraction. The velocity of a sound beam in the incident medium is less than that in the transmitted medium, causing the beam to be bent away from the normal ($\theta_i < \theta_t$).

wavelength is called Rayleigh scattering. Red blood cells act as Rayleigh scatterers in Doppler ultrasound. *Rayleigh scatterers have strong frequency dependence (f^2 to f^6).*

Reflectivity

Many factors influence the fraction of incident intensity that is reflected at an interface toward the transducer—the acoustic impedance mismatch, the angle of incidence, the size of the structure compared with the wavelength, the shape of the structure, and the texture of the surface of the interface. The combination of these factors is described by the term reflectivity.

Differences in reflectivity are partially responsible for the patient-to-patient variations that sonographers observe when performing a particular type of examination. Ultrasound imaging systems are capable of detecting extremely small changes in reflectivity, on the order of one in a million.

Refraction

If the ultrasound beam strikes an interface between two media at an incident angle of 0 degrees (normal incidence), a fraction of the incident intensity is reflected back to the first medium and the rest is transmitted into the second medium without a change in direction. If the beam strikes the interface at an angle other than 0 degrees, however, the transmitted part is refracted or bent away from the projected straight-line path (Figure 1-11). This change in direction as the ultrasound beam crosses a boundary is called refraction.

A similar effect caused by the refraction of light is seen when an object under water is viewed from above. If one reaches for the object through the water, the spatial inaccuracy becomes immediately apparent. Refraction may contribute to the misregistration of an object depicted in the sonographic image.

Refraction of sound waves obeys Snell's law, which relates the angle of transmission to the relative velocities of sound in the two media. (Note that this relationship is not based on acoustic impedance.) If the acoustic velocity in the first medium is less than that in the second medium, then the angle of transmittance is bent away from the normal as illustrated in Figure 1-11. For example, this occurs at a tissue-bone interface. If the acoustic velocity in the first medium is greater than that in the second medium, then the angle of transmittance bends toward the normal from the expected straight-line path. If the acoustic velocity is the same in the two media, no refraction (bending) occurs, although the acoustic impedances may be different. Nor does refraction occur at normal incidence, regardless of the relative velocities in the two media.

Divergence

A sound wave, if not impeded, will spread out in all directions (called divergence) as the wave propagates from the sound source. The rate of divergence increases as the size (diameter) of the sound source decreases.

Interference

Sound waves demonstrate interference phenomena or the superposition of waves (algebraic summation). As an example of interference, consider the ripple patterns produced in the water when three swimmers dive into a pool one after the other from three different diving boards located along the side of the pool. If the entries are separated in time then each diver produces a characteristic ripple pattern. If all three divers reenter the water simultaneously, then the resulting complex ripple pattern consisting of large and small water disturbances is a combination of the three individual patterns.

If waves with the same frequency are in phase, they undergo constructive interference. Waves are in phase if crossing and inflection points are matched along the distance or time axis (Figure 1-12). Constructive interference results in an increased amplitude.

If waves with the same frequency are out of phase, they undergo destructive interference; that is, a decrease in amplitude results because the peaks are not matched in the same position (Figure 1-13). Completely destructive interference occurs when the waves are of the same frequency and amplitude and are completely out of phase (i.e., the trough of one wave corresponds to the peak of the other). The result is a wave with zero amplitude; hence, the summation wave disappears. The effect of one wave is countered by the opposite effect of the other wave. For example, when two opposing players approach a soccer ball, the player who kicks it first controls the direction of travel. If both players kick the ball simultaneously with equal force, the applied

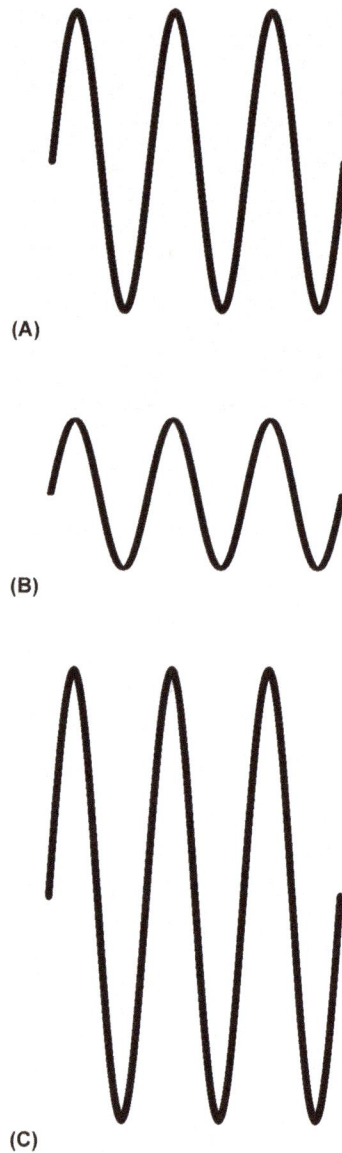

(A)

(B)

(C)

FIGURE 1-12. Constructive interference or superposition (algebraic summation) of waves. (**C**) the resultant wave with increased amplitude, is the sum of waves (**A** and **B**).

forces cancel each other and the ball does not move toward either goal.

Every combination—from completely constructive to completely destructive interference—can occur, resulting in a complex wave summation. Figure 1-14 shows the result when waves with differing

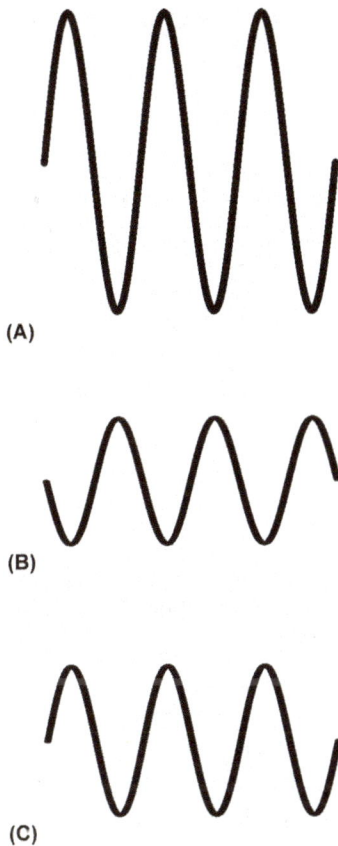

(A)

(B)

(C)

FIGURE 1-13. Destructive interference. (**C**) the resultant wave with decreased amplitude, is the sum of waves (**A** and **B**) which are out of phase.

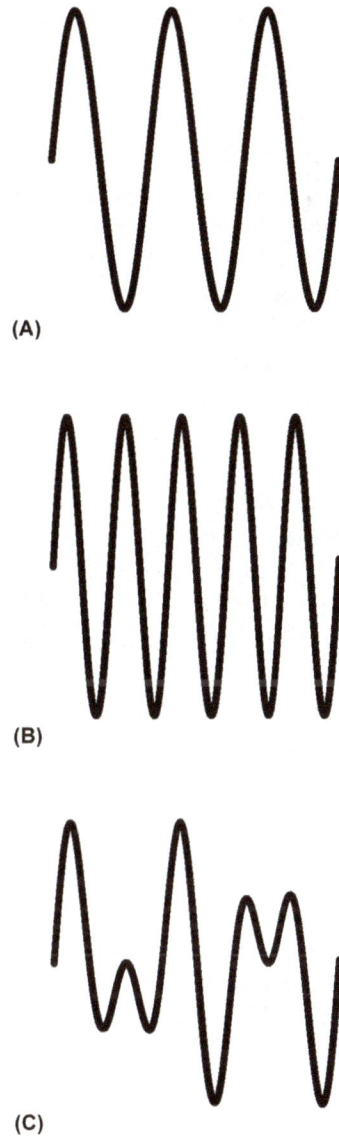

(A)

(B)

(C)

FIGURE 1-14. Complex wave interference. (**C**) is the summation of two waves (**A** and **B**) with slightly different frequencies.

frequencies create interference. Interference plays an important role throughout sonography, including pulse transmission, electronic focusing, and Doppler velocity measurement.

Absorption

Absorption is the only process whereby sound energy is dissipated in a medium, primarily in the form of heat. Once energy is transferred from ultrasound to the medium, it cannot be recovered and intensity is reduced. All other modes of interactions (reflection, refraction, scattering, and divergence) decrease the ultrasonic beam intensity by redirecting the energy of the beam.

The absorption of an ultrasonic beam is related to the viscosity and elasticity of the medium, but is strongly dependent on the frequency of the wave. The ability of molecules to move past one another characterizes the viscosity of a medium; high viscosity provides great resistance to molecular flow. For instance, a low-viscosity fluid (water) flows more freely than a viscous one (maple syrup). The frictional forces must be overcome by vibrating molecules, and thus more heat is produced in the viscous maple syrup.

If the frequency is increased, the molecules must move more often, thereby generating more heat from the drag caused by friction (viscosity). Also, as the frequency is increased, less time is available for the molecules to recover during the relaxation process. Molecules remain in motion, and more energy is necessary to stop and redirect them, again producing more absorption. *The rate of absorption is directly related to the frequency*. If the frequency doubles, the rate of absorption also doubles.

Consider the mechanical action of rubbing one's hands together. The movement produces heat. If the hands are rubbed together more rapidly (higher frequency), increased warming occurs. If lotion is placed between the palms so the resistance is decreased (lower viscosity), less heat is generated.

The peak amplitude of acoustic pressure decreases as the wave propagates through a homogeneous medium (Figure 1-15). Absorption is enhanced if the frequency is increased (Figure 1-16).

Attenuation

Attenuation includes the effects of both scattering and absorption in the reduction of intensity as the ultrasound wave propagates through a medium. *The rate of attenuation depends on the medium and frequency of the ultrasound wave*. To a first approximation, the rate of attenuation increases linearly with frequency.

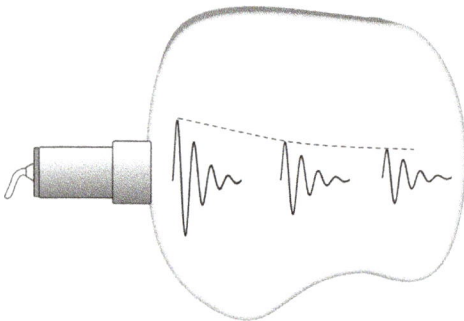

FIGURE 1-15. Attenuation of acoustic energy as a sound beam propagates through the medium. The decrease of the peak acoustic pressure is denoted by the dashed curve.

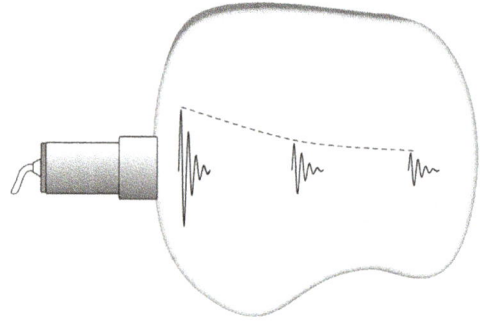

FIGURE 1-16. Attenuation of acoustic energy as a high-frequency sound beam propagates through the medium. The decrease of the peak acoustic pressure is denoted by the dashed curve. Compared with Figure 1-15, the frequency is increased; consequently, the rate of energy loss is more rapid.

Values for the fractional intensity remaining after transmission through different media (1 cm in thickness) at a frequency of 1 MHz are listed in Table 1-5. Ultrasound readily passes through blood, whereas bone and lung are strong attenuators.

As frequency is increased, the reduction of the ultrasound intensity with distance becomes more pronounced. This has a practical consequence in medical imaging. The ultrasound beam and returning

TABLE 1-5 • Loss of Intensity by Attenuation in Different Tissues	
Medium	**Remaining Intensity after 1-cm Path (%)***
Blood	96
Fat	87
Soft tissue	85
Skull	1
Lung	0.01
Water	99.95

*Frequency is 1 MHz

echoes that form the image must travel through tissue. *The depth of penetration becomes less as frequency is increased—the ability to observe deep-lying structures is forfeited (Figure 1-17).*

Decibel

Although no standard reference intensity for ultrasound has been established, a useful method for determining the intensity is to make relative measurements that compare the value at one point with a reference intensity. The following analogy may help illustrate the concept: Johnny owns 25 marbles, Tommy 50. To find out how much Johnny's marbles weigh in ounces, we place them on a scale. If we are interested only in the relative weight of Johnny's marbles, we say they are "half as heavy as Tommy's." The absolute weight in ounces is not known but the relative weight can be described with respect to a standard (Tommy's marbles).

Relative intensity measurements are usually made and given in decibels (dB).

As a rule of thumb, 3 dB corresponds to an intensity change of a factor of 2. Therefore, an intensity loss of 12 dB means that the intensity has been reduced by a factor of 16 (12 dB divided by 3 dB is four and 2^4 yields 16).

Penetration

High-frequency sound waves are attenuated more rapidly than low-frequency sound waves. Thus, the ability to penetrate tissue is reduced at higher frequencies. In addition, a reflector positioned at progressively greater depths generates progressively lower-intensity returning echoes. Intensity attenuation factors for human tissues are usually stated at a frequency of 1 MHz (Table 1-6). The attenuation rate at frequencies above 1 MHz is estimated by assuming that the attenuation rate is directly proportional to the frequency. For

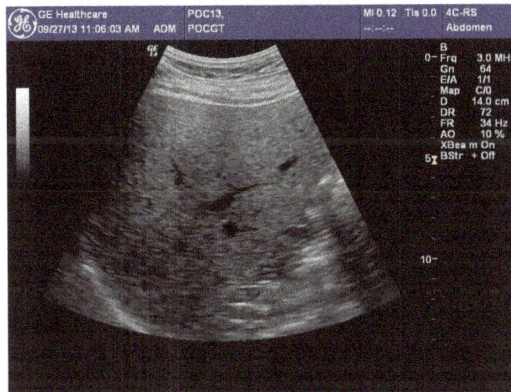

(A)

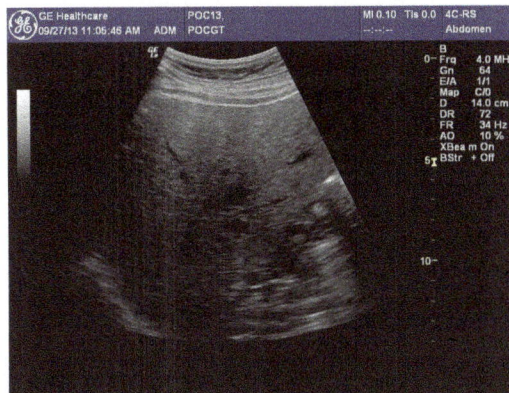

(B)

FIGURE 1-17. Effect of frequency on penetration. (**A**) The depth of penetration for 3 MHz center frequency is greater than 12 cm in an abdominal scan. (**B**) The depth of penetration for 4 MHz center frequency is 7 cm for the same patient.

TABLE 1-6 • Attenuation Rates for Different Media	
Material	**Attenuation Rate (dB/cm-MHz)**
Blood	0.18
Fat	0.6
Soft tissue average	0.5–0.8
Liver	0.5
Muscle	1.2
Skull	20
Lung	40
Water	0.002

example, the attenuation rate at 4 MHz for fat is calculated by multiplying 4 MHz times 0.6 dB/(cm-MHz). The result is 2.4 dB/cm for fat when the frequency is 4 MHz.

ECHO RANGING

A system that can generate an ultrasonic pulsed wave and detect the reflected echo after a measured time permits the distance to an interface (i.e., the depth of the interface) to be determined. This technique is called echo ranging, a concept that formed the basis of sonar developed during World War II.

In diagnostic ultrasound, reflections of the sound beam from interfaces along the ultrasonic path are of primary interest. A pulsed ultrasound wave is transmitted into the body, strikes an interface (acoustic mismatch between two media), and is partially reflected to the transducer, as determined by the reflection coefficient. The successive echoes arising from the various acoustic impedance mismatches along the path result in ultrasonic detection of reflectors within the body.

The average velocity of ultrasound in tissue is 1540 m/s. For an interface exactly 1 cm away, the total time for the sound wave to travel out to the interface and back to the transducer is 13 μs (Figure 1-18). The distance to an interface is indicated by the elapsed time; in other words, the time of travel to and from the interface at a constant velocity is governed by the distance of travel. As the depth to the interface

increases, the elapsed time increases. For an interface 10 cm away, 130 μs between the transmitted pulse and the returning echo is required.

For echo ranging to delineate the position of an interface accurately, certain conditions must hold: *(1) the ultrasound wave must travel directly to the interface and back to the transducer along a straight-line path and (2) the velocity of sound must remain constant along the path of travel.*

ECHO INTENSITY

In ultrasound imaging, the transducer sends out a pulsed wave and subsequently detects the returning echo. Intensity loss occurs by attenuation of the transmitted wave going out to the interface and also by attenuation of the reflected wave coming back toward the transducer from the interface. The rate of attenuation depends on tissue type and frequency. The intensity of the detected echo from an interface is diminished by increasing the distance of travel.

In general, absorption is a major contributor to the overall intensity loss. *Structures with the same reflectivity are not always depicted with the same signal level because of differences in path length (effect of attenuation).* The presence of a cyst (low attenuation) or gallstone (high attenuation) along the beam path alters the displayed signal level distal to these structures (Figures 1-19 and 1-20).

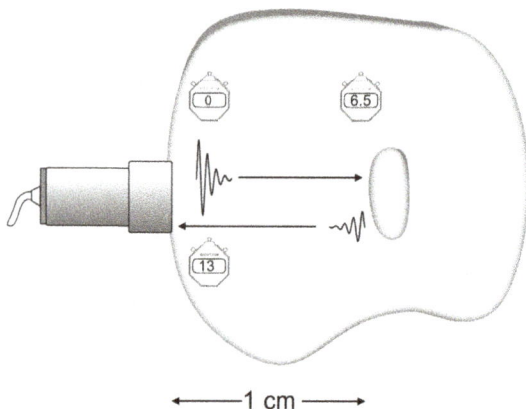

FIGURE 1-18. Echo ranging. For a reflector at a depth of 1 cm, the time after transmission at which the echo is received is 13 μs, assuming a constant acoustic velocity of 1540 m/s.

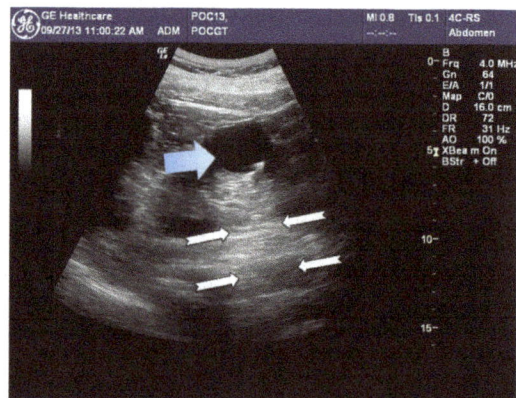

FIGURE 1-19. Sonogram of a kidney with a cyst. The liquid-filled structure has a low rate of attenuation (large arrow) causing acoustic enhancement distal to the cyst (small arrows).

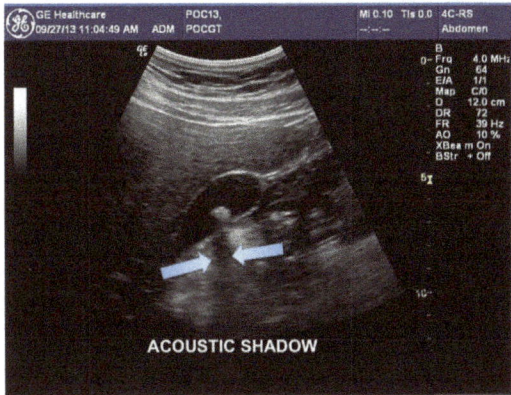

FIGURE 1-20. Sonogram of a gallbladder with gallstones. The crystalline structures have a high rate of attenuation causing acoustic shadowing distal to the gallstones (arrows).

References

Hedrick WR: Technology for diagnostic sonography, St. Louis, 2013, Elsevier.

Hedrick WR, Hykes DL, Starchman DE: Ultrasound physics and instrumentation, ed 4, St. Louis, 2005, Elsevier.

Kremkau FW: Diagnostic ultrasound: principles and instruments, ed 8, Philadelphia, 2011, WB Saunders.

Zagzebski JA: Essentials of ultrasound physics, St Louis, 1996, Mosby-Year Book.

2

Real-Time Image Formation

OBJECTIVES

- To describe the important design features of an ultrasound transducer.
- To list the parameters that characterize pulsed-wave operation.

- To understand real-time image formation.
- To recognize the advantages and limitations of B-mode imaging.

KEY TERMS

Bandwidth
Center frequency
Field of view
Frame rate
Lead zirconate titanate (PZT)
Line of sight
Piezoelectric effect

Pulse duration
Pulse repetition frequency
Scan converter
Scan line
Scan line density
Scan range
Spatial pulse length

TRANSDUCER DESIGN

A transducer is any device that transforms one kind of energy into another (e.g., mechanical to electrical). The ultrasound transducer must perform two functions—transmit an ultrasound wave by electrical stimulation and then convert the detected echo into an electrical signal for processing and display.

The sonographic information content depends on the transmitted beam characteristics, which in turn are governed by the transducer. Design criteria for ultrasound transmission with an imaging transducer include frequency in the megahertz range, pulsed-wave operation, directional control, regulated intensity, and limited spatial extent (beam width and spatial pulse length). For positional information utilizing the echo-ranging principle, a short burst is required and thus the sound beam must be turned on and off rapidly. A unidirectional beam with limited physical dimensions is crucial to identify the location of the reflector with spatial accuracy. Small beam width and spatial pulse length (related to frequency) restricts the region in which the echo could have been formed. To compose a two-dimensional image, transmitted pulses must be directed along different anatomic paths. This is accomplished by scanning, sweeping, or steering the beam automatically and very rapidly throughout the field of view. Uniform intensity is desirable so that structures with similar reflectivity produce echoes of similar strength regardless of location within the scanned volume. Although some manipulation of intensity is possible, uniform ultrasonic fields cannot be obtained in practice.

In echo detection, mechanical vibrations induced in the transducer generate the electric signal. If a Chinese gong is allowed to move only once after being struck and then cushioned with a pillow to shorten the duration of the vibration, a single-cycle sound wave will be produced. The transmitted wave would move out to some distant object, undergo reflection, and then return toward the source. In such circumstances, the echo incident on the transducer is also a single-cycle vibration. Since the position of any object in space can be determined only to an accuracy of about one-half wavelength, a spatial resolution limit is imposed by wavelength. The ability to distinguish two objects separated by a small distance along the direction of propagation is called axial resolution. Because frequency and wavelength are inversely related, short wavelengths, which produce finer spatial detail, correspond to high frequencies.

If one wavelength is a good approximation of the smallest detectable object, what frequency is required for a resolution of 1 mm in tissue? In nature, bats and porpoises generate ultrasound with a frequency of around 100 kHz or a wavelength of 1.54 cm. Thus, this frequency is too low to provide the desired spatial detail. Frequencies above 1.5 MHz are necessary to generate waves with wavelengths less than 1 mm. For medical diagnostic sonography, it is evident that the operating frequency must be in the megahertz range.

PIEZOELECTRIC PROPERTIES

The transducer must be manufactured, since nothing in nature can be readily adapted to transmit ultrasonic waves in the megahertz frequency range. The construction of a high-frequency transducer relies on a phenomenon known as the piezoelectric effect (characterized as the accumulation of an electric charge by a material in response to mechanical stress). Piezoelectric crystals have regions of positive and negative charge on each molecule (called dipoles), although often the dipoles are randomly distributed. Aligning the dipoles in a well-defined pattern is accomplished by applying an electric field to the heated crystal during fabrication. Once cooled, the molecules continue to maintain their alignment. *Ultrasound transducers should not be autoclaved, because the dipoles become randomly oriented at high temperature, resulting in a loss of piezoelectric properties.*

The molecular configuration of the dipolar molecules in piezoelectric materials is responsible for their unique properties. Electrodes are placed on the opposite faces of the crystal. When a voltage is applied, the molecules twist to align themselves with the electrical field (positive molecules toward the negative electrode, negative molecules toward the positive electrode), thereby thickening the crystal (Figure 2-1). If the plates are reversed in polarity, the molecules twist back in the opposite direction, reducing the crystal thickness. Alternating polarity causes expansion and contraction of the crystal, which creates mechanical vibrations. When the expanding and contracting crystal is placed in contact with the skin, sound waves are transmitted into the body. Electrical stimulation of the crystal controls the generation of the ultrasound beam by the transducer (rapid on and off switching).

A piezoelectric crystal can also act as a receiver by converting mechanical vibrations induced by the incident ultrasonic echo into voltage variations. Electrical signals from multiple echoes, separated in time, are processed and ultimately displayed.

(A)

(B)

(C)

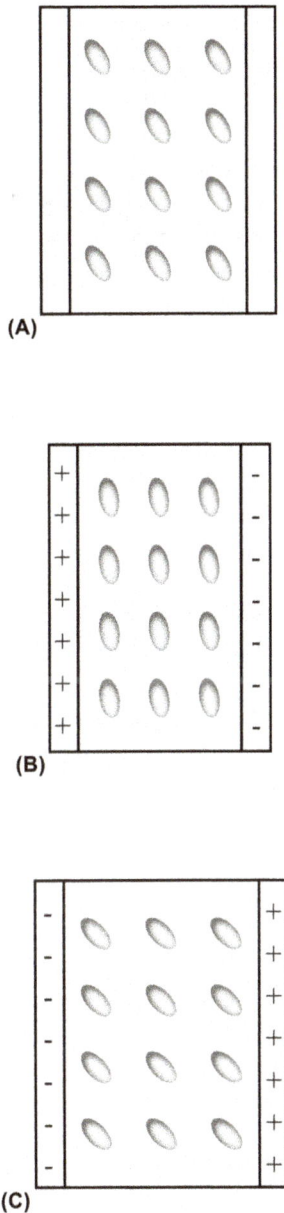

FIGURE 2-1. Crystal response when voltage is applied to the excitation electrodes. (**A**) Normal thickness when no electrical field is applied. (**B**) Contraction of the crystal caused by rotation of dipoles in which the positive region of each dipole (shown in darker gray) moves closer to negative plate. (**C**) Expansion of the crystal caused by rotation of the dipoles in which the positive region on dipole moves closer to negative plate. The polarity is reversed from that depicted in B.

Frequency does not change when the ultrasound wave enters one medium from another. The same frequency generated by the transducer is transmitted into the patient. However, a change in wavelength occurs between the crystal and the tissue caused by velocity differences in the two media (1540 m/s for tissue and approximately 4000 m/s for the crystal).

PIEZOELECTRIC MATERIALS

The transducer material almost universally used in sonography is lead zirconate titanate (PZT). PZT represents a family of piezoelectric ceramics with various additives, which alter crystal characteristics to match a particular application. PZT has the desirable properties of efficient energy conversion, proper frequency range, and ability to be molded in a particular size and shape. These ceramics are brittle and easily broken if dropped.

TRANSDUCER CONSTRUCTION

The major component of a transducer is the piezoelectric crystal with thin, metal electrodes plated on two opposed crystal surfaces to create voltage polarity. To improve the transfer of energy to and from the patient, the matching layer is placed in contact with the crystal along the transmitted beam path. The matching layer provides an intermediate step-down in acoustic impedance from the crystal to the body, allowing for more efficient energy transfer. Most current transducers utilize multiple matching layers with even smaller increments of impedance, resulting in very efficient transfer of the sound energy into the body. Crystal ringing is diminished by the introduction of backing material on the opposite side from the matching layer. The entire crystal assembly, including the electrodes, matching layer(s), and backing material, is housed in an electrically insulating plastic case. To reduce the electromagnetic interference, a radiofrequency shield composed of a hollow metallic cylinder is placed around the crystal and backing material and electronically grounded to the front electrode surface. An acoustic insulator, made of rubber or cork, coats the inner surface of the radio-frequency shield to prevent the transmission of ultrasound energy into the plastic housing.

PULSED-WAVE OUTPUT

In echo-ranging systems, the transducer must pause after sound transmission to "listen" for the returning echoes. Because the crystal cannot send and receive simultaneously, pulsed-wave transmission occurs after an appropriate listening time has elapsed (Figure 2-2). The inactive transmission period (time in receiving mode) determines the maximum depth for reflector placement, which is called the scan range. The excitation voltage waveform is a short burst consisting of one to three cycles with a frequency equal to the desired center frequency.

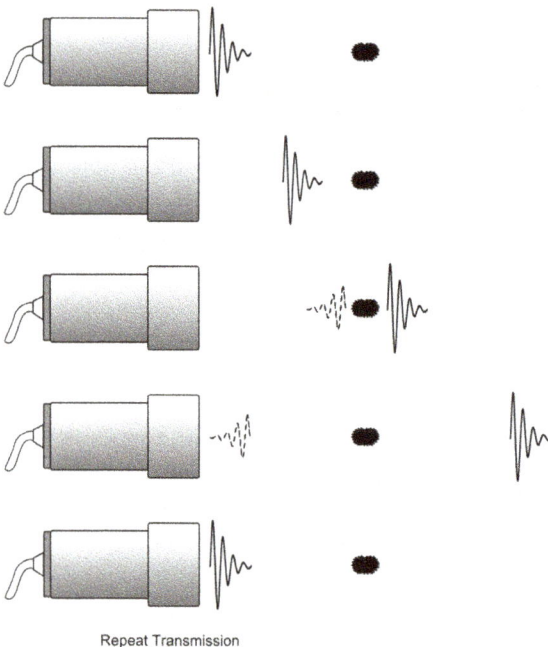

Repeat Transmission

FIGURE 2-2. Time sequence of the transmission/listen cycle. The transducer actively generates a four-cycle pulse of short duration (solid line), which subsequently moves away from the transducer into tissue and creates an echo (dotted line) from a single reflector along the path. During the listen time interval, the transmitted pulsed wave continues to propagate along the directed path as the echo returns to the transducer and is detected prior to the next transmitted pulse.

Pulse Repetition Frequency

The number of times the crystal is electrically stimulated per second to produce the pulsed-wave output is called the pulse repetition frequency. The maximum pulse repetition frequency depends on the scan range. If the scan range is increased, the maximum pulsed-wave transmission rate is reduced since more time is required for the sound wave to travel the longer distance. Patient ALARA considerations and transducer heating often dictate that the transmission rate is less than the maximum pulse repetition frequency for a given set of conditions. In designing their systems, manufacturers usually vary the pulse repetition frequency with the scan range. A single, independent control for pulse repetition frequency is normally not available to the operator.

Spatial Pulse Length

Ideally, for each pulse, a short packet of ultrasound energy of the appropriate frequency (i.e., 5 MHz for a 5-MHz transducer) is directed into the body. In practice, the pulse is composed of a range of different frequencies that encompass the labeled operating frequency. The operating frequency, also called the center frequency, represents the most dominant frequency in the transmitted pulse. The physical extent of this short-duration wave (distance along the direction of propagation at one instant in time) is called the spatial pulse length and equals the product of the center frequency wavelength and the number of cycles in the pulse. For example, spatial pulse length is 0.9 mm for a transducer with a center frequency of 5 MHz (corresponding to a wavelength of 0.31 mm) that transmits a pulse that is three cycles in duration.

For good axial resolution, a small spatial pulse length is necessary. To shorten the pulse spatially, the number of cycles must be reduced or the frequency must be increased to decrease wavelength.

Pulse Duration

The pulse duration, or temporal pulse length, is the time interval for one complete transmitted pulsed wave. Pulse duration corresponds to the actual time of active ultrasonic generation by the transducer. The effectiveness of the matching layer to transfer the energy into tissue and the ability of the backing material to quickly dampen the pulse affect the pulse duration. The pulse duration is the product of the number of cycles in the pulse and the period of the wave. The three-cycle pulse from a 5-MHz transducer has a spatial pulse length of 0.9 mm with a pulse duration of 0.6 μs. A decrease in spatial pulse length corresponds with shorter pulse duration. If the pulse from a 5-MHz transducer is reduced to two cycles, then the spatial pulse length is 0.6 mm with a pulse duration of 0.4 μs.

Duty Factor

Typical B-mode scanner operation with a pulse duration of less than 1 μs and a pulse repetition frequency of 1 kHz transmits ultrasound only 0.1% of the time. Most of the time (99.9%), the transducer is operating in receive mode. The duty factor is the fraction of time ultrasound generation is active and is calculated as the ratio of the pulse duration and the pulse repetition period.

Bandwidth

Continuous output transmits a wave with a single frequency. *For pulsed-wave output, however, because of the complex nature of the short-duration transmission, multiple frequencies are present.* Waves with different frequencies combine by interference to form the transmitted waveform. The frequency distribution (plot of the fraction of the output with a certain frequency versus frequency) shows a centrally peaked spectrum, with the center frequency having the greatest amplitude (Figure 2-3). The frequency bandwidth is a measure of the range of frequencies present in the transmitted pulse.

Pulse duration and bandwidth are inversely related. In diagnostic ultrasound imaging, transducers with broad bandwidths are desirable because both ultrasound transmission and detection can be enhanced. The bandwidth for a 5-MHz transducer bandwidth may extend from 3 to 7 MHz.

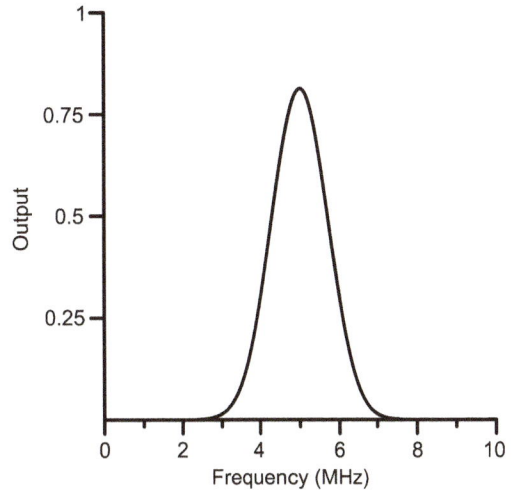

FIGURE 2-3. Frequency distribution of the transmitted pulse. The dominant component in the transmitted output (5 MHz for this distribution) is the center frequency.

FOCUSING

Divergence causes a decrease in the intensity as the beam propagates away from the transducer. This is easily understood by considering that the emitted energy is distributed over a larger and larger area. The intensity incident on a reflector is reduced as the distance between the reflector and the transducer increases. The reflected beam also diverges during return to the transducer and, thus, creates a partial "miss" of the ultrasound wave at the transducer (Figure 2-4).

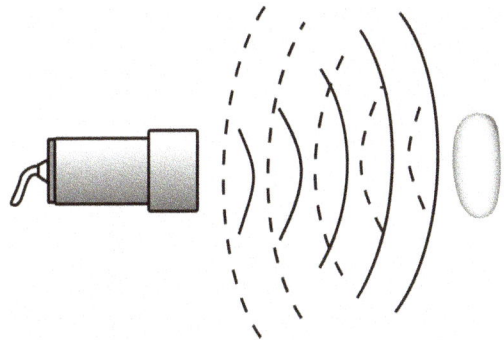

FIGURE 2-4. Divergence of the sound wave causes reduced intensity in both transmitted (solid lines) and received (dashed lines) directions.

Divergence is responsible for intensity loss during transmission and echo detection. Also, spatial registration of the reflector is compromised by the widening wavefront.

The transmitted waves can be directed to converge at a specific point. This manipulation, called focusing, narrows the beam width and raises the intensity over a small area at a specific distance from the transducer. Compared with a nonfocused beam, the focused beam produces a stronger echo whose spatial origin can be more accurately determined. This is true only for structures within the focal zone of the transducer, however, where beam width is most narrow. Focusing techniques and the resulting ultrasonic fields are discussed in the next chapter.

COMPOSITE PIEZOELECTRIC MATERIALS

A composite transducer element is formed by dicing the piezoelectric material into an array of regularly spaced, rectangular pillars and filling the interspace with epoxy resin. The composite material has a very wide bandwidth, high sensitivity, low acoustic impedance, and is easily shaped for the desired configuration for geometric focusing. Most modern transducers are manufactured with composite piezoelectric materials.

PRINCIPLES OF REAL-TIME IMAGING

Real-time B-mode imaging depicts the reflectivity of structures and continually updates this information for display by repeating the data acquisition process. Each new updated image is a frame. The two-dimensional frames are formed rapidly and shown in succession with a customary frame rate of 15–35 frames per second. Real-time imaging can be compared with other dynamic modalities (motion picture films) in which a series of stop-action shots is taken and then viewed rapidly one after another to depict motion. Or, if the transducer is being moved, the anatomy within the changing scan plane is shown.

The displayed image is continuously and rapidly updated with new echo data as a narrow, pulsed beam is repeatedly directed throughout the field of view. Field of view is the anatomical region interrogated by scanning the ultrasound beam. The depth of the field of view is the scan range along the direction of propagation. The width of the field of view is the lateral extent over which the beam is scanned. Various brightness levels or shades of gray depict the relative reflectivities of structures. The transducer can be moved to any scan plane without any restriction in movement (the transducer is not mounted on a scanning arm). Instant feedback with respect to anatomical structures detected within the field of view facilitates sonographic procedures. The major disadvantage of B-mode imaging is that the relatively small field of view makes anatomical identification difficult or excludes nearby structures from the image.

Data collection for each frame is a combination of echo ranging and directional beam scanning. The time delay between the transmitted pulse and the received echo determines the distance of the reflector from the transducer in the scan direction. A series of echoes following the transmitted pulse allows placement of multiple reflectors encountered by the beam along the anatomic path. Only those structures that lie along the direction of propagation within the beam are interrogated. This linear sampling according to the beam path is called line of sight or scan line. An image is composed of multiple scan lines by acquiring echo-ranging data along different sampling directions. Each scan line is acquired sequentially in the scanning progression (Figure 2-5). Displayed brightness for a reflector is controlled by the intensity of the detected echo.

A pulsed-wave, narrow beam is first directed along a well-defined path, and after the echoes are received, the ultrasound beam is then shifted to a new sampling direction. Beam orientation is controlled by electronic means in a repetitive, automated fashion without intervention by the operator. Multiple scan lines, sampled in sequence, throughout the field of view forms a single image. Every scan line requires one transmit pulse to interrogate interfaces along the directed path. This scanning process is repeated to produce successive images of the anatomic structures within the field of view.

(A)

(B)

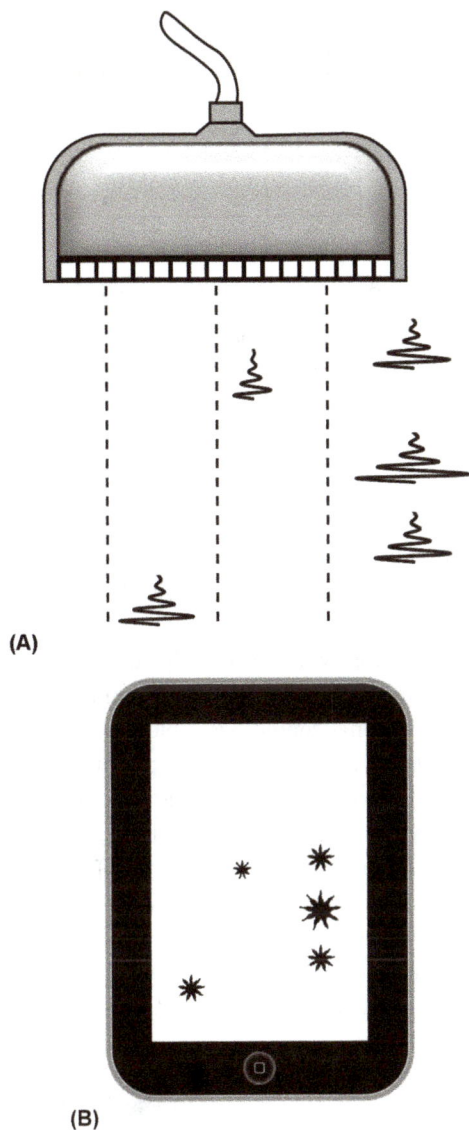

FIGURE 2-5. Image formation in real-time ultrasound. (**A**) Echo-ranging data from three scan lines acquired sequentially allows spatial mapping of the detected echoes. The origin and amplitude of each echo along the respective beam paths (dashed lines) are shown. (**B**) Image display on the monitor in which the brightness of the dot represents the signal level of the detected echo. The placement of each dot depends on the scan direction and echo-ranging applied to each detected echo.

As motion becomes more rapid within the field of view, a faster frame rate is necessary to display the structures without jerkiness. The time for the pulse to travel to the depth of interest and back to the transducer—along with the need for good spatial detail provided by a large number of scan lines in each image—imposes a restriction on the frame rate. Commonly 120–150 scan lines compose noncardiac image with rates of 15–30 frames per second.

SCAN CONVERTER

Scan lines form the building blocks for each image. Each scan line represents activation of a group of crystals in the transducer array, which is established by the scanning format. The ultrasound beam is directed into the patient in a well-defined pattern. Hence, no external reference is necessary to determine the location of each scan line. A digital scan converter assembles the echo-induced signals from each scan line and then deciphers this information during readout into the two-dimensional image for display. The digital representation of signal levels allows image processing to enhance presentation of the echo data.

Analog-to-Digital Conversion

The information content of the echo-induced signals must be changed to a digital format for the write/read functions of the scan converter. The translation process is called analog-to-digital conversion and is dependent upon the number of bits available in the digitization process. Some accuracy is sacrificed when a signal is digitized, as occurs in the translation of information from the detection system (signal amplitude and spatial location of the reflector) to a form that is understood by the computer (0s and 1s). In sonography, the analog signal is a voltage waveform generated by the crystal in response to mechanical stress induced by the echo. Increased voltage corresponds to higher signal strength. Ultimately, the bit depth of the analog-to-digital converter affects both contrast and dynamic range of the sonographic image.

Spatial Representation

The information obtained from a scanned area is divided into small, square picture elements called pixels, which are combined to form the image (similar to pieces of a jigsaw puzzle). Each pixel corresponds to a unique location within the field of view, designated by spatial coordinates, and is associated with the signal strength from tissue at that location. The amplitude of the received signal is transformed to a number by the analog-to-digital converter before placement in the scan converter. The number of pixels available depends on the matrix size, which denotes the number of rows and columns in the pictorial representation. For example, a 750 × 350 matrix has 750 rows and 350 columns. The image is composed of a total of 262,500 individual pixels (the number of rows multiplied by the number of columns).

To place the digitized echo-induced signal in the correct pixel within the image matrix, the spatial coordinates (row and column) must be specified. The time to echo detection in conjunction with the known transmitted beam path accomplishes this task. A composite picture of all scan data is formed as signal levels along successive scan lines are registered in the matrix format of the scan converter. Figure 2-6 shows two scan lines within the field of view in which three reflectors with varying signal strength are detected. The signal amplitudes are represented by the appropriate pixels in an 8 × 8 matrix (Figure 2-7).

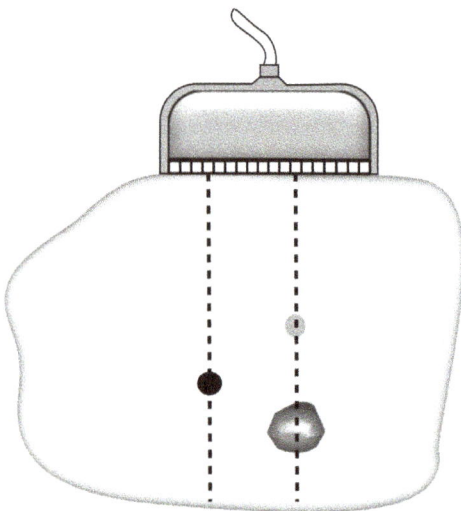

FIGURE 2-7. An 8 × 8 matrix depicting the structures observed in Figure 2-6. The pixels corresponding to the three reflectors are assigned different values based on the amplitude of the received echoes.

The spatial coordinates dictate the position within the matrix and the numerical value of the pixel represents the signal level. In this example, the pixels, corresponding to the various reflectors, are assigned different values based on the amplitude of the echoes.

To display the array of numerical signal values on the monitor, while technically correct, would be extremely difficult to understand. Communication of the informational content via a picture with varying gray levels is a far easier format to comprehend. Each pixel is depicted as a uniform shade of gray based on the pixel value and a lookup table that translates pixel value to brightness (gray-scale map). The distribution of the shades of gray among all pixels composes the image (Figure 2-8). Each pixel is depicted as a single shade, because only one value is stored in scan converter for that pixel. The same value is assumed

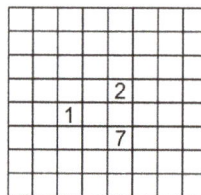

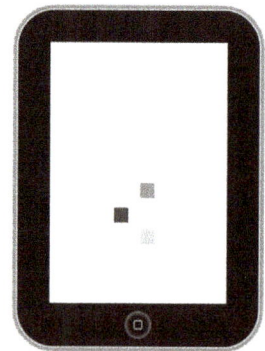

FIGURE 2-6. Two scan lines illustrate sampling along different paths. Note that the two reflectors are detected along the one scan line.

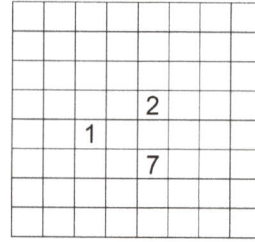

FIGURE 2-8. Signal level for each pixel in the image matrix is converted to gray level for display (only three pixels are shown for illustration purposes). Gray levels from black to light gray represent increasing echo amplitude.

to exist throughout the spatial extent represented by the pixel. This assumption is most appropriate for pixels with small physical dimensions. Once more, some accuracy is lost by the digital representation of spatial location. As the matrix size increases (more pixels), the system has the potential for better spatial detail, which is demonstrated by the digitized photographs of a mountain scene with varying matrix sizes (Figure 2-9). Currently, matrix size for B-mode imaging is 350×750, 480×640, 600×800, or

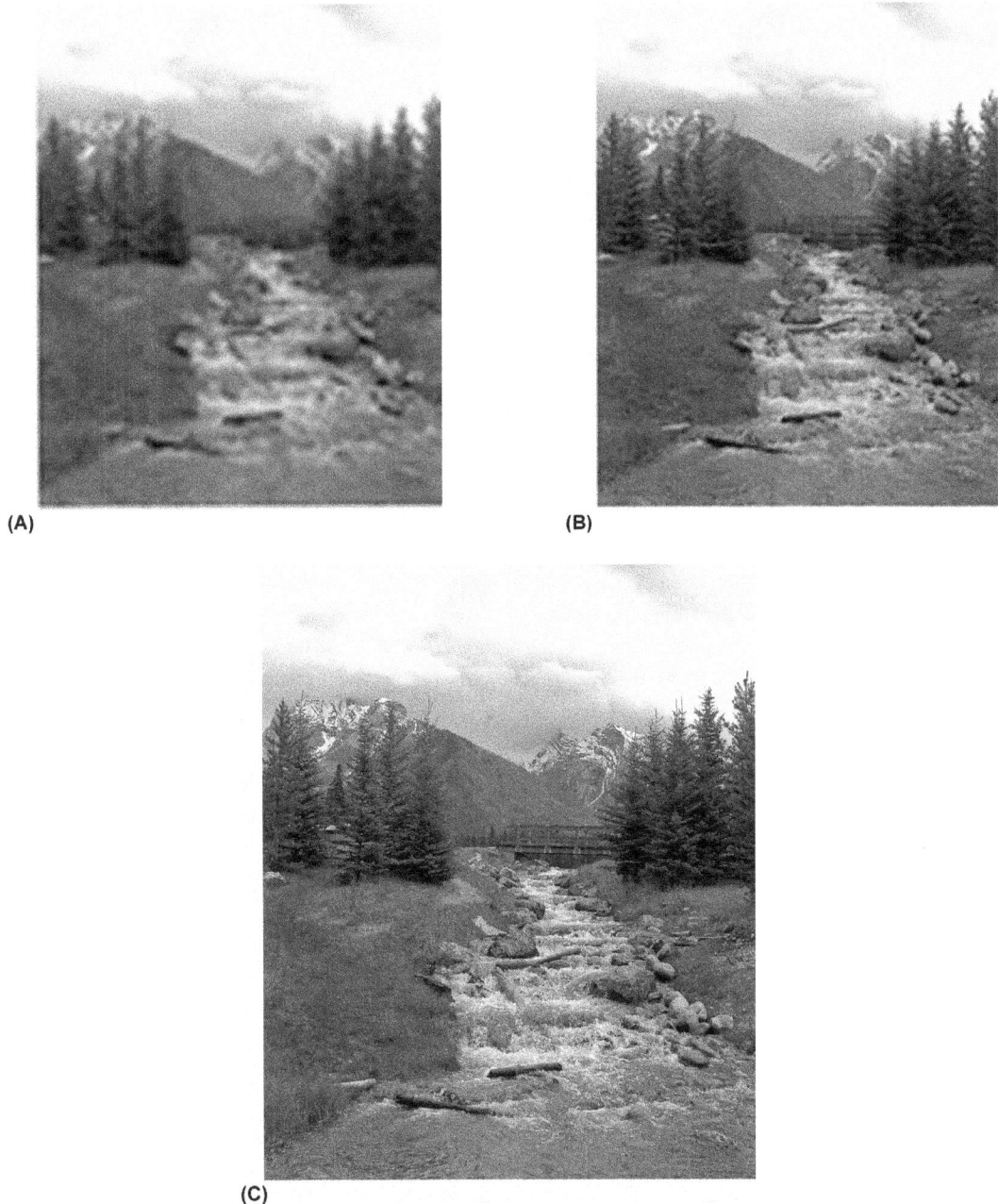

(A)

(B)

(C)

FIGURE 2-9. Matrix representation of a mountain scene to demonstrate the effect of pixel size. (**A**) 100×80; (**B**) 200×160; (**C**) 2500×2000.

720 × 960 depending on manufacturer and model. At a viewing distance of 18 in from the monitor, the individual pixel elements are not distinguished, and the image appears spatially continuous.

IMAGE DISPLAY

Solid-state flat panels such as liquid crystal displays have become the preferred display monitor for most applications. The screen is divided into pixels similar to the scan converter matrix that holds image information. The light level or color for each screen pixel is individually controlled. Computer monitors have higher spatial resolution and frame rates than available using a commercial TV video signal.

The video interface converts the digital image to an analog format for video transmission. Each pixel in a row of the image matrix is read sequentially left to right to form one video line. After the readout for one row is completed, the pixels in the next row are then read sequentially to form another video line. This row-by-row readout sequence continues such that a video line is formed for each row in the image matrix. Data obtained for a video line in the image matrix are shown as one brightness-modulated line across the screen. The brightness of light on the screen is dictated by the level of the input signal (stored pixel value), and the position is governed by the readout scanning sequence. Because readout of the image matrix and line-by-line scanning of the screen are synchronized, the signal level in the image matrix—and therefore the echo measurements—is converted into a visual image. The refresh rate for computer monitors is 60–120 times each second.

TIME CONSIDERATIONS

In conventional B-mode, one transmitted pulse is required for each scan line. A finite amount of time is necessary for the pulsed wave to probe the full extent of the scan range and then return as an echo to the transducer (13 μs for every centimeter of tissue). This sequence of events must be repeated for every scan line. Extending the scan range requires increased

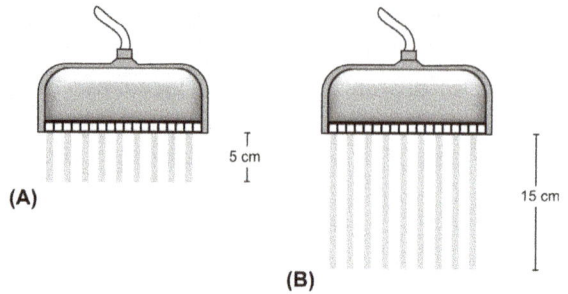

FIGURE 2-10. Time to acquire a scan line depends on scan range. (**A**) A 5-cm scan range requires 65 μs for each scan line. (**B**) A 15-cm scan range requires 195 μs for each scan line.

measurement time to acquire the echo-ranging data for each scan line (Figure 2-10).

The following analogy illustrates the concept of image formation in real-time ultrasound. A company wants to determine the effectiveness of advertising in attracting customers to its stores. Imagine that three stores are each located one block away from a central starting point in the directions of north, east, and west. A sonography student, who is also an employee of the company, is assigned to monitor the number of customers in each store and then report these findings. The student walks east to the first store, counts the customers, and returns to the starting point where the information is recorded. Other stores are evaluated sequentially in the same manner. However, customer number is only accurate for the time at which the observation occurred. Customers will enter and leave a store. To obtain the current status and demonstrate changes in activity, the student must return to each store repeatedly.

In this analogy, the number of customers indicates the reflectivity of the interface, and the directions east, north, and west represent different beam paths (a total of three scan lines). Obviously, customer data are not obtained instantaneously; travel time to and from each store limits the rate at which the information can be collected.

By constraining the sonography student to walk at a constant velocity along the straight-line paths, the time required to obtain customer data from all stores is well defined. Similarly, the acoustic velocity in soft tissue is finite (and assumed constant) and imposes a restriction on the frequency of sampling. The scan range for the stores is set at one block. However, if the stores were located farther away, then the sonography student must travel a longer distance, and the information updates would be less frequent. As scan range is increased, more time must be allotted to accumulate data for a scan line. Compare the total time to collect an image consisting of eight scan lines for the different scan ranges shown in Figure 2-10. The total acquisition time for a scan range of 5 cm is 520 μs but increases to 1560 μs for a scan range of 15 cm.

Frame Rate Limitations

Since a finite amount of time is necessary to form one image, the number of frames that can be acquired and displayed each second (frame rate) is limited. The maximum frame rate depends on the scan range and the number of scan lines per frame. If the scanning depth and/or number of lines of sight are increased, the maximum frame rate must decrease. The number of frames per second is ultimately limited by the rate of travel (acoustic velocity in tissue, 1540 m/s).

For instance, assume that the field of view is set to a depth of 10 cm. The data collection time for each scan line is 130 μs. If 100 lines of sight compose each image, then the maximum frame rate becomes 77 frames per second. Extending the scan depth reduces maximum frame rate. If 100 scan lines are to be maintained for a change in scan range from 10 to 20 cm, the maximum frame rate is decreased to 38 frames per second. Table 2-1 demonstrates the relationship between the number of scan lines, the depth of scanning, and the maximum frame rate. The time required for data collection for each frame equals the reciprocal of the maximum frame rate.

The number of scan lines per frame and pulse repetition frequency determine the actual frame rate, which is often less than the maximum frame rate. B-mode scanners usually operate at pulse repetition frequencies between 2000 and 5000 Hz but can be as high as 12,000 Hz to preserve lateral resolution while maintaining a high frame rate. Some sacrifice in scanning depth may be required at higher pulse repetition

TABLE 2-1 • Maximum Frame Rate versus Depth and the Number of Scan Lines

Depth (cm)	100 Lines	150 Lines	200 Lines
5	154	103	77
10	77	51	38
15	51	34	26
20	38	25	19
25	30	20	15
30	25	17	12

frequencies. The manufacturer sets the frame rate, scan range, field of view, and number of scan lines based on the clinical application. These default values are likely to produce reasonable image quality for the average patient. Several approaches are possible to compensate for an increase in scan depth. The real-time unit may automatically decrease the frame rate but maintain the same number of scan lines. On the other hand, both frame rate and number of scan lines may be adjusted downward. The number of scan lines may be reduced without a loss in resolution by narrowing the field of view. Often, several transducers with different center frequencies are available for use with a single ultrasound unit. Each frequency is optimized with respect to the number of scan lines and frame rate as a function of sampling depth according to the clinical application.

Temporal Resolution

As motion becomes more rapid within the field of view, a faster frame rate is necessary to display the structures without jerkiness. The finite transit time for the ultrasound pulse to travel to the depth of interest and back to the transducer, as well as the need for good spatial resolution provided by a large number of scan lines in each image, imposes a restriction on the frame rate.

Often, spatial resolution is sacrificed to improve the temporal resolution of fast-moving structures.

BEAM WIDTH

The design criteria for an imaging transducer include directional beam transmission with a narrow beam width. These characteristics are desirable, because small objects can be scanned individually and distinguished as separate entities.

A single object smaller than the beam width produces an echo whenever it is intercepted by the beam. An echo is created regardless of the lateral position of the object in the ultrasonic field (Figure 2-11). The lateral dimension of the object in the image is defined as the same size as the beam width. Multiple small objects displaced laterally but equidistant from the transducer are not resolved when encompassed by the broad beam (Figure 2-12). Remember, axial displacement of reflectors is detected by altered echo times. Multiple samplings with successive narrow beams enable the objects to be observed as separate entities (Figure 2-13).

Sampling by the transmitted pulse is restricted laterally by the width of the beam. Objects located outside the beam do not contribute signals for that scan line. Scanning with a narrow beam width throughout

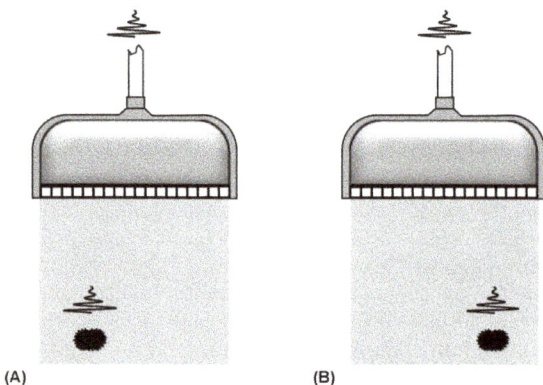

FIGURE 2-12. Generation of echoes by two identical, small objects within the ultrasonic field using a broad beam (gray region). Since the depth is the same and the echoes arrive at the transducer simultaneously, the presence of two structures is not discernible in the induced signal. The signal strength is twice that in Figure 2-11.

the field of view enables an accurate depiction of interrogated structures in the lateral direction.

LATERAL RESOLUTION

Lateral resolution describes the ability to distinguish two objects adjacent to each other that are perpendicular to the beam axis. Decreasing the beam width improves the lateral resolution by allowing objects close together to be sampled individually. Scan line density is the number of scan lines per distance or angular arc distributed across the field of view. *The line density also affects lateral resolution.* High scan line density improves the detection of small reflectors and provides more accurate presentation of boundary shapes.

Returning to the analogy involving the student sonographer, suppose, instead of three stores in the survey, numerous stores are distributed throughout

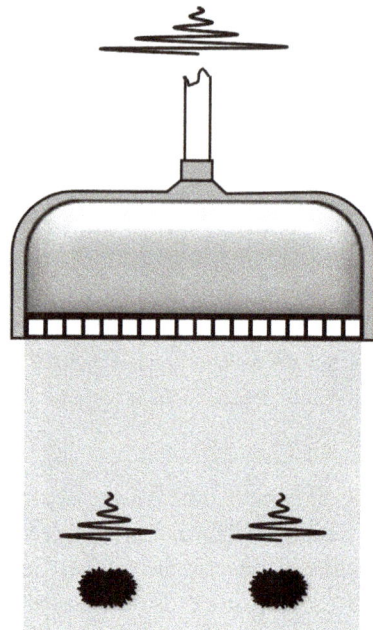

(A)   (B)

FIGURE 2-11. Generation of an echo by small object within the ultrasonic field using a broad beam (gray region). (**A** and **B**) At the constant depth, regardless of lateral location in the broad beam, the measured time for induced signal from this single reflector is the same.

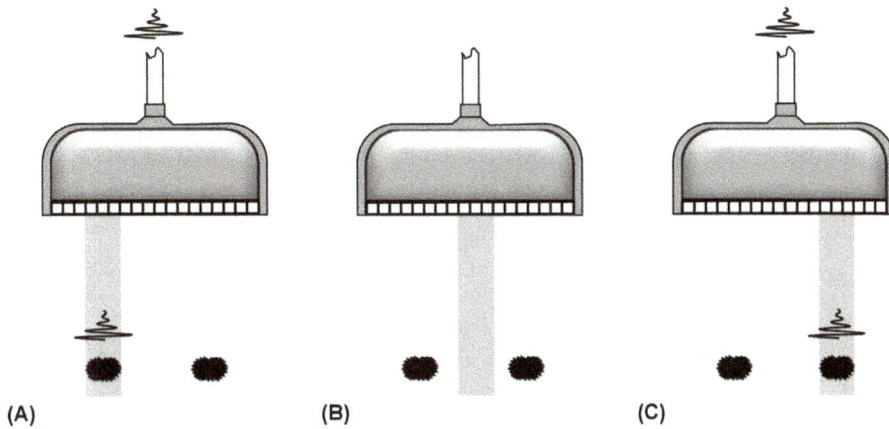

FIGURE 2-13. By reducing the beam width and collecting echo-range data along multiple scan lines (three separate gray regions) separated in time, the induced signal indicates both depth and the lateral position of the reflector. (**A**, **B**, and **C**) Time sequence for signals received along different beam paths enables the two reflectors to be resolved.

the city. If travel is restricted to the directions of north, east, and west, then only stores located along these three paths are encountered—other stores are missed. To include all stores in the survey, the student sonographer must walk in many different directions. For real-time image formation, increasing the number of scan lines improves the spatial sampling throughout the field of view. The effect of line density on image quality is illustrated in Figures 2-14-2-16.

In practice, lateral resolution deteriorates when the separation between two scan lines is greater than the beam width. Reducing the number of scan lines to achieve a high frame rate sometimes creates this situation. Furthermore, if the scan range and the

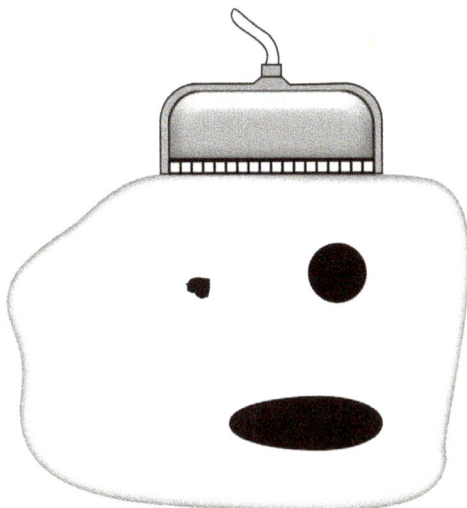

FIGURE 2-14. Scan volume containing three reflectors. Each object has a unique size and shape.

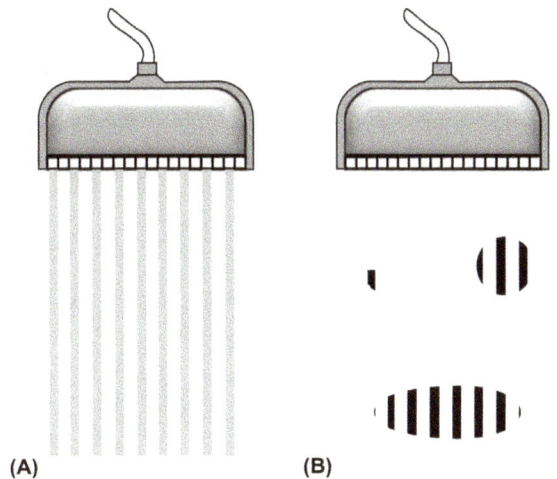

FIGURE 2-15. Effect of low scan line density on lateral resolution. (**A**) Sampling by scan lines (total of eight denoted by gray regions). (**B**) Image formed by scanning the reflectors in Figure 2-14 along the scan lines in A. Border for each reflector is poorly defined. Small objects may not be observed, because low scan line density creates sampling voids within the field of view.

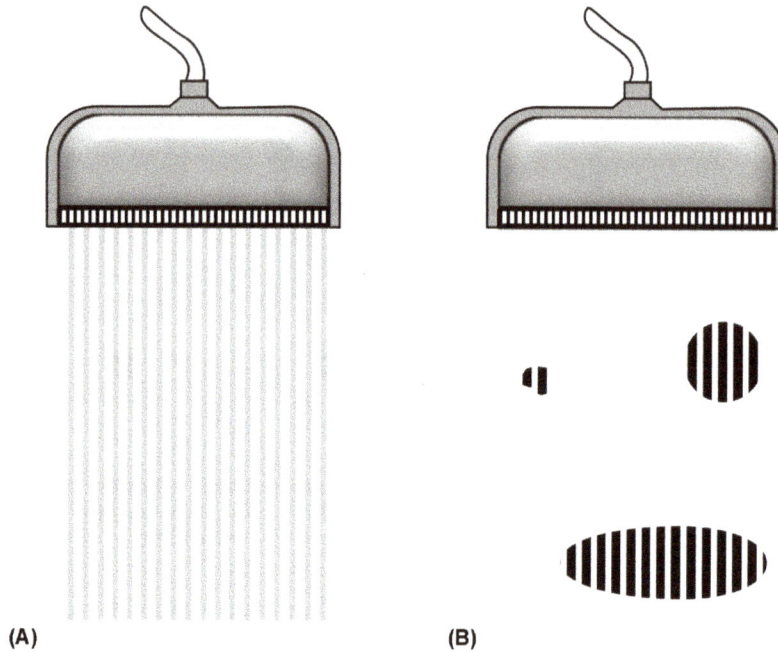

FIGURE 2-16. Lateral resolution is improved by increasing scan line density. (**A**) Sampling by scan lines (total of 18 denoted by gray regions). (**B**) Image formed by scanning the reflectors in Figure 2-14 along the scan lines in A. Increased scan line density improves the border definition of the reflectors.

pulse repetition frequency are unchanged, expanding the width of the field of view decreases the scan line density. Extending the scan range, while maintaining the frame rate and the width of the field of view, has a similar effect (reduced scan line density).

References

Hedrick WR: Technology for diagnostic sonography, St. Louis, 2013, Elsevier.

Hedrick WR, Hykes DL: Image Formation in Real-Time Ultrasound. Journal of Diagnostic Medical Sonography 11, 246–251, 1995.

Hedrick WR, Hykes DL, Starchman DE: Ultrasound physics and instrumentation, ed 4, St. Louis, 2005, Elsevier.

Kremkau FW: Diagnostic ultrasound: principles and instruments, ed 8, Philadelphia, 2011, WB Saunders.

Zagzebski JA: Essentials of ultrasound physics, St Louis, 1996, Mosby-Year Book.

3

Transducers

OBJECTIVES

- To describe the various types of ultrasound transducers.
- To understand the principle of electronic focusing with multiple-element arrays.
- To comprehend spatial sampling in three dimensions with a focused, pulsed beam.

KEY TERMS

Channel
Curvilinear array
Dynamic receive focusing
Electronic focusing
Linear array

Phased array (sector)
Slice thickness
Steered linear array
Vector array

TRANSDUCER TYPES

Classification of real-time transducers is based on the method by which the ultrasound beam is focused and directed through the field of view. Each transducer type produces a unique image format. Multiple-element transducers, including linear array, curvilinear array, phased array, and vector array, form and scan the beam electronically. This assortment of transducers, while requiring appropriate selection by the operator for a particular clinical examination, enables optimal sonographic information content.

LINEAR ARRAY

A linear array contains 150–300 small, rectangular crystals arranged side by side along a straight row. The crystals are electronically and independently controlled to activate ultrasound transmission and then to detect the incident echoes for data collection. Each element with the associated electronics for transmission and reception constitutes a channel. In the most simple scheme, the crystals are excited in a sequential fashion to form the individual scan lines (Figure 3-1). The number of crystals in the array

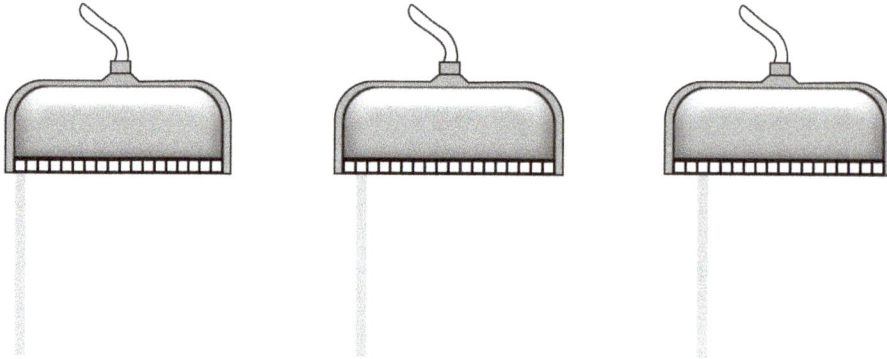

FIGURE 3-1. Beam scanning with a linear array. The beam direction is determined by element selection during transmission. Three scan lines are shown. Sweeping the beam across the entire field of view is accomplished by stimulating each element in sequence.

determines the maximum number of scan lines for each image. If the array contains 150 individual crystals that are stimulated one at a time in sequence, 150 scan lines can be acquired.

The first crystal in the array is excited, and then a time delay for collection of the echoes from reflectors along that path is imposed before the next crystal is activated. The duration of the delay is set by the scan range (13 μs is required for every centimeter of depth). For example, assume that a maximum viewing depth of 15 cm is desired. The first crystal is electronically stimulated to produce an ultrasound beam, and 195 μs later the second crystal is excited. After another 195 μs, the third crystal transmits a pulsed wave. This cycle of excite-delay-excite continues until all 150 crystals have been activated in turn and the corresponding echoes detected to form one image. The same timed activation sequence for the crystals in the array is repeated for the next image. The time required to collect scan data for one image is set by the scan range and the number of scan lines, which establishes the maximum frame rate. The 15 cm scan range limits the pulse repetition frequency to 5133 pulses per second. With 150 lines per frame, the maximum frame rate is 34 frames per second.

The size of the crystal (radiating surface) dictates the physical dimensions of the ultrasonic field. A major problem with the above described method is that small crystal size produces a short, narrow

ultrasonic field near the transducer, which then diverges rapidly. Larger radiating surface extends the depth before divergence, but results in increased beam width near the transducer (Figure 3-2). When multiple small crystals are stimulated as a group, the respective ultrasonic fields from all crystals act in concert to provide a more favorable beam pattern by maintaining beam width over an extended range (Figure 3-3). This scheme, however, while superior to a small, single crystal acting alone, creates fewer scan lines for the same scan plane width, which causes a loss in spatial detail. For example, assume that the individual crystals are fired in groups of

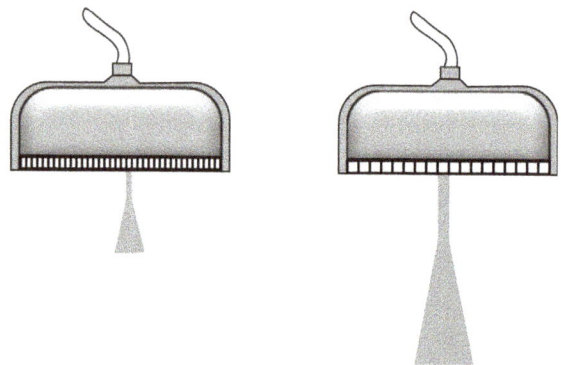

FIGURE 3-2. Crystal size in the transducer array affects the beam pattern. Small crystals create a narrow beam width near the transducer that rapidly diverges. Large crystals produce a wider beam width with less rapid divergence.

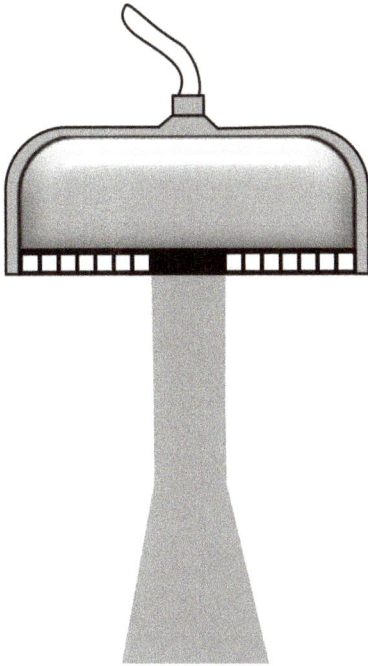

FIGURE 3-3. A group of small crystals activated simultaneously creates an ultrasonic field that corresponds with the size radiating surface (similar to a single large crystal).

four. By using adjacent blocks of four crystals, four scan lines that are spaced widely apart can be created (Figure 3-4). Although beam width at increased depth is more narrow, line density is very low.

To achieve good spatial definition throughout the field of view, a combination of narrow beam width and high line density is achieved by incrementing the multiple-element crystal group by one element. Figure 3-5 shows the transmission sequence for the first three scan lines for a linear array in which crystals 1 through 4 are stimulated and then after the time delay for echo detection crystals 2 through 5 are excited. After another listen period, crystals 3 through 6 are activated. In other words, a set of four crystals is fired as a group to produce the desired beam pattern and, by overlapping groups, the number of scan lines is maximized. This approach produces high scan line density, since the radiating surface for each transmitted beam is incremented by one crystal element. The array must

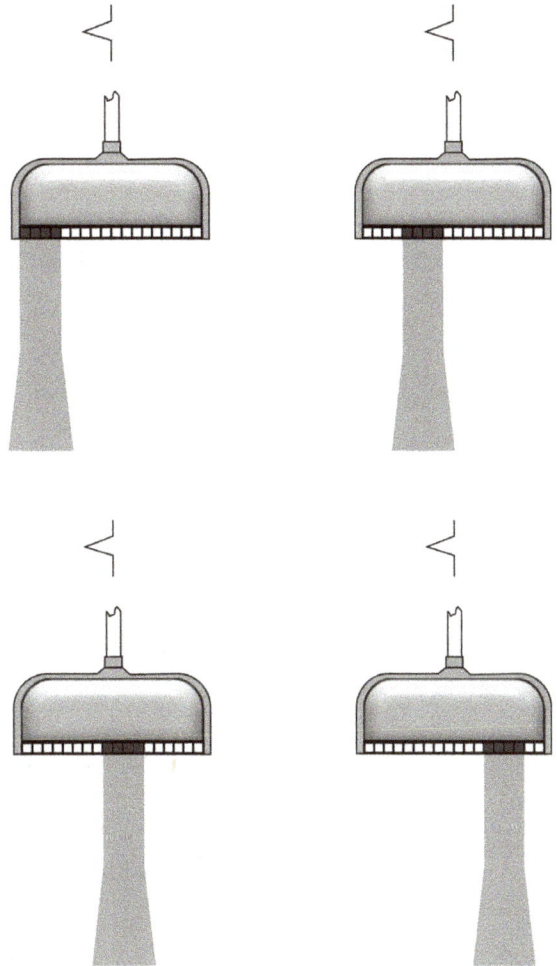

FIGURE 3-4. Four elements comprise a group, and the group is shifted by four elements for each successive transmission. In this scheme, four scan lines across the field of view are produced.

contain multiple, small crystals which are individually controlled to implement this technique.

The multiple-element linear array produces good temporal resolution (high frame rate) and good spatial resolution (beam width and number of scan lines). The field of view is presented in a rectangular format, with the in-plane width equal to the physical length of the row of crystals. Figure 3-6 illustrates the orientation of the parallel scan lines with respect to the transducer. The linear array has a flat face, which causes difficulty in maintaining transducer-patient contact when a wide

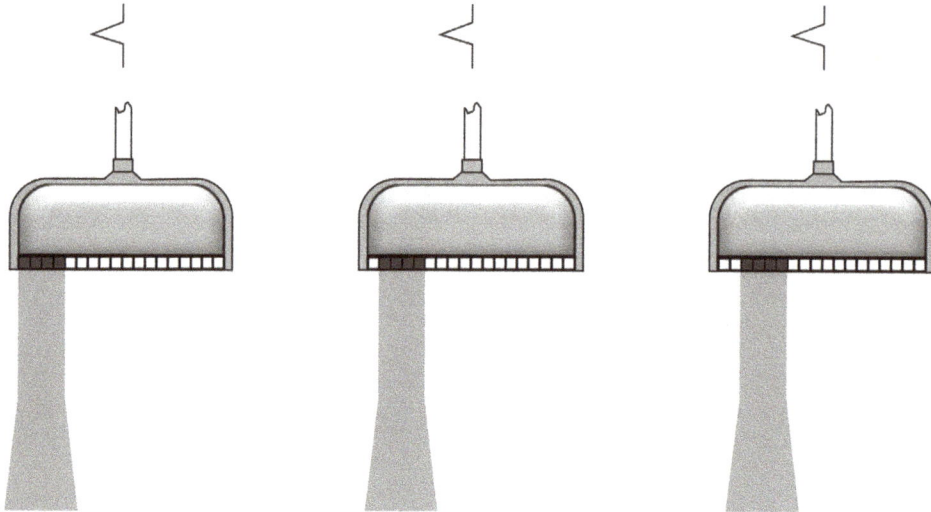

FIGURE 3-5. Beam sweeping with a linear array. Four elements compose a group, and the group is shifted by one element for each successive transmission. Scan line density is increased by overlapping segments.

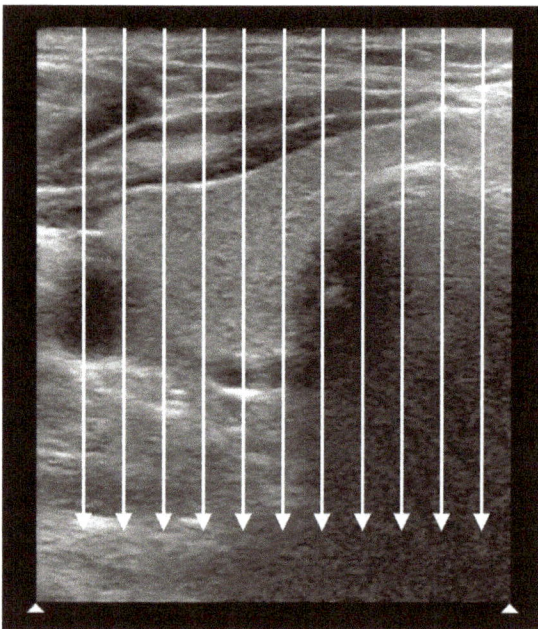

FIGURE 3-6. The direction and orientation of scan lines shown for an image obtained with a linear array transducer.

field of view is desired. Nevertheless, this step-down technique improved the image quality of real-time scanners dramatically, although additional adjustments in focusing are necessary to narrow the beam width further so the spatial detail can be optimized.

ELECTRONIC FOCUSING

Regardless of whether a single crystal or a group of crystals is excited, the rectangular shaped radiating surface creates an ultrasonic field with beam dimensions equal to the aperture close to the transducer face (Figure 3-7). However, the ultrasonic field for a linear array is not symmetrical, and therefore the beam width along the row of crystals (in-plane) and perpendicular to the row of crystals (elevation) must be specified

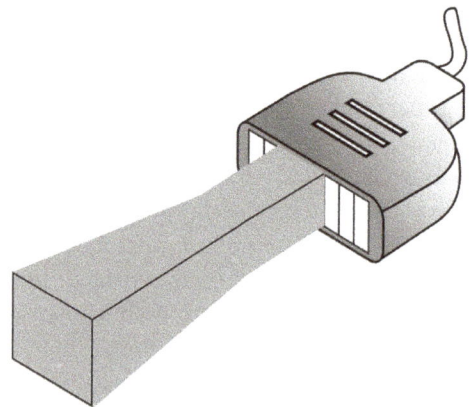

FIGURE 3-7. Beam pattern produced by a group of crystals in the linear array in the absence of focusing. Beam width in the elevation and in-plane directions are shown.

separately. Ultrasound beams are focused to reduce the beam width and to increase intensity, which in turn improves spatial resolution and sensitivity. Focal length is the distance from the transducer to the point of focus and focal zone describes the region near the focal point where the beam width is most narrow.

Focusing is applied in two directions (in-plane as well as elevation) to narrow the beam width perpendicular to the direction of propagation. Along the in-plane direction, focusing is accomplished electronically to vary the depth of focus and to narrow the beam width to about 1 mm within the focal zone. Mechanical focusing along the elevation direction determines the thickness of tissue represented by the cross-sectional image (referred to as slice thickness) and is accomplished either by curving the crystal or, more commonly, by placing an acoustic lens in front of the crystal. The beam is most narrow at a specified depth, which is established by the lens or curvature of the crystal. Focusing in the elevation direction is applied equally to each crystal. The slice thickness is not constant along the scan line but is typically 3–5 mm within the fixed focal zone.

Focusing Dynamics

The excitation sequence of one group of crystals followed by the next group prohibits mechanical focusing of the ultrasound beam in the in-plane direction. The relative position of a crystal in the group dictates the focusing requirements for that crystal. *Because crystals in the array belong to multiple firing groups, the focusing requirements change and cannot be achieved by static mechanical means.* For example, crystal 3 is the center of a five-crystal firing sequence involving crystals 1 through 5, the second position for crystal group 2 through 6, and the first position for crystal group 3 through 7. This changing position dictates different focusing requirements for that crystal and thus prohibits fixed mechanical focusing in the in-plane direction.

Fortunately, linear arrays are electronically focused in the in-plane direction (Figure 3-8), which (when combined with mechanical focusing in the elevation direction) creates a narrow beam within the matched focal zones (Figure 3-9). Focusing in the in-plane direction can be adjusted to any depth along the scan

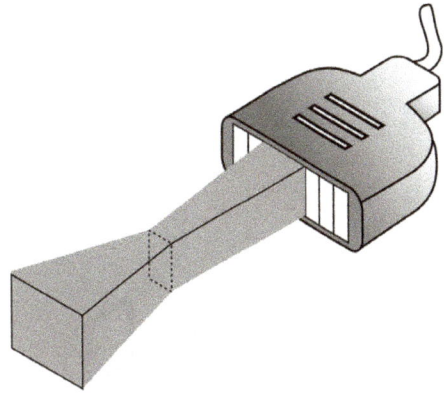

FIGURE 3-8. Electronic focusing of an array reduces the beam width in the in-plane direction near the point of focus.

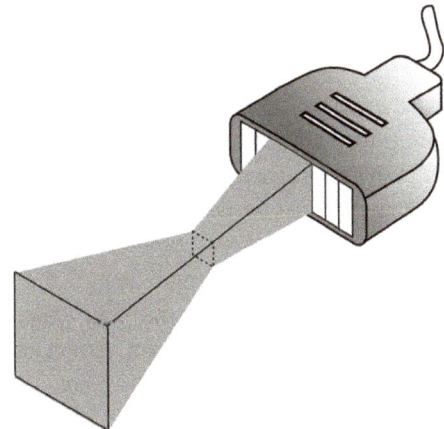

FIGURE 3-9. Resultant beam pattern when both mechanical focusing and electronic focusing are applied. Note the reduced beam width in the elevation direction (thinner slice thickness) compared with Figure 3-8.

line, whereas the beam width in the elevation direction is not changeable. The spatial sampling volume has axial, lateral, and slice thickness components (Figure 3-10).

Principle of Focusing

Electronic focusing involves the interference (algebraic summation) of ultrasound waves from multiple crystals separated in time and space. Each crystal produces a particular wave pattern, and the overall pattern derived from a group of crystals is the summation of all the wave patterns from the individual crystals (Huygens' principle). The main beam axis is centered at the middle

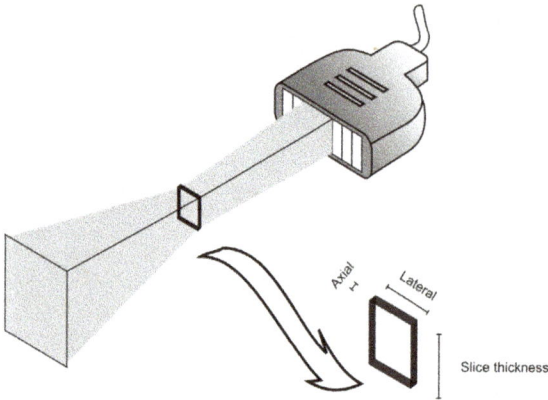

FIGURE 3-10. Instantaneous spatial sampling for the pulsed beam within the ultrasonic field. In-plane focusing affects lateral beam width. Mechanical focusing in the elevation direction determines the slice thickness. Spatial pulse length controls the axial extent of the pulsed wave.

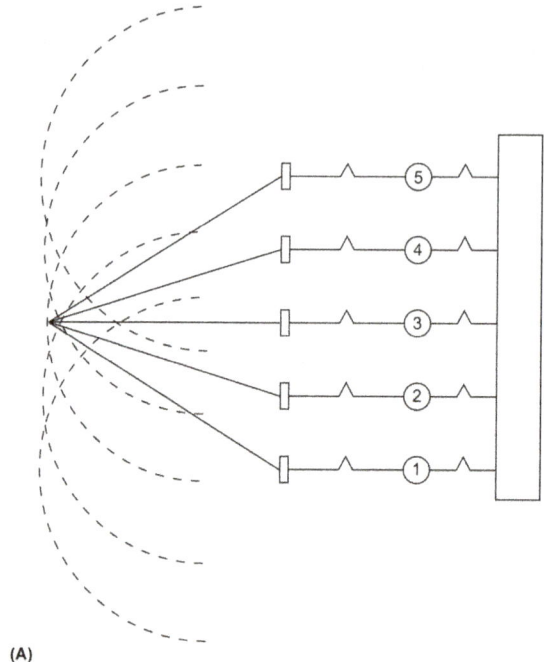

(A)

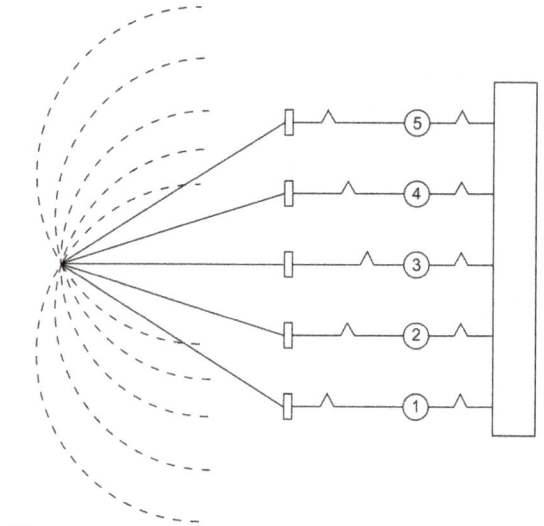

(B)

crystal in the group. Electronic focusing is accomplished by altering the activation order of crystals by well-defined time delays. These delays are small compared with the time required for the sound beam to travel to the depth of interest. The exact timing depends on the crystal position and the focal length desired. The wavefronts generated by all crystals in the group are made to arrive at a specific point (focal point) simultaneously, and the result is a focused beam at that point.

Figure 3-11 demonstrates electronic focusing for beam transmission using five crystals. The positions of the crystals are arranged so the distance from crystal 1 to the point of interest is greater than the distance from crystal 2 to that same point. And the pathway from crystal 3 to the point of interest has the shortest distance compared with all other crystals in the group. Crystals 1 and 5 are equidistant to the point of interest (similarly, crystals 2 and 4 are also matched in distance to the point of interest). The wavefronts from each of the five crystals must arrive at the focal point at exactly the same time. This is accomplished by exciting crystals 1 and 5 first, delaying a short time before exciting crystals 2 and 4, and finally waiting another short time before exciting crystal 3. The ultrasound beam is thus focused in the in-plane direction, producing a narrow beam width over a limited depth near the focal point. The next segment of crystals (2 through 6) is fired in the same manner (2 and

FIGURE 3-11. Electronic transmit focusing. **(A)** If five crystals are stimulated at the same time, the wavefronts do not arrive simultaneously at the desired point, because all crystals are not equidistance to that point. **(B)** Transmit delay lines excite the crystals at slightly different times. The wavefronts arrive simultaneously at the desired point, and the result is a focused beam. Crystals 1 and 5 are stimulated first, then 2 and 4, and then 3. Changing the time delays allows focus point to be placed at different depths.

6, 3 and 5, then 4) to produce another similarly focused beam, but directed along a different scan line. The remaining segments across the array are also focused by this delayed activation technique. A beam with a set focal length is swept through the field of view to collect echo data for an image. Improved spatial detail (lateral resolution) is thus obtained within the focal zone corresponding to a particular depth in the image.

Transmit Focusing

Transmit focusing allows one of several possible focal lengths within the scan plane to be designated. *The depth of the transmit focal zone is altered by adjusting the delay times between crystal excitations.* If the specified depth of focus does not correspond to the region of interest, a new focal zone depth may be selected (by modifying the delay line timing) to rescan the field of view. Electronic control of the elements allows focusing to different depths along the scan line, which, in turn, narrows beam width in the in-plane direction within the selected focal zone (Figure 3-12).

High scan line density images with multiple, transmit focal zones throughout the scan range are also possible. Each scan line is divided into segments corresponding to the number of focal zones. Multiple transmitted beams, each with a focal length matched for a particular segment, must sample each scan line. Multizone transmit focusing typically slows the frame rate, because data must be acquired for all the scan lines across the array with one focal length before the acquisition is repeated with a different focal zone depth. For example, assume that the unit can be focused at three different depths for the same "image." In reality, three separate scan line collections, each with a particular focal length, must be obtained before they are combined into one "final image" for viewing. Since each scan line is interrogated multiple times to compose each real-time image, frame rate is reduced significantly.

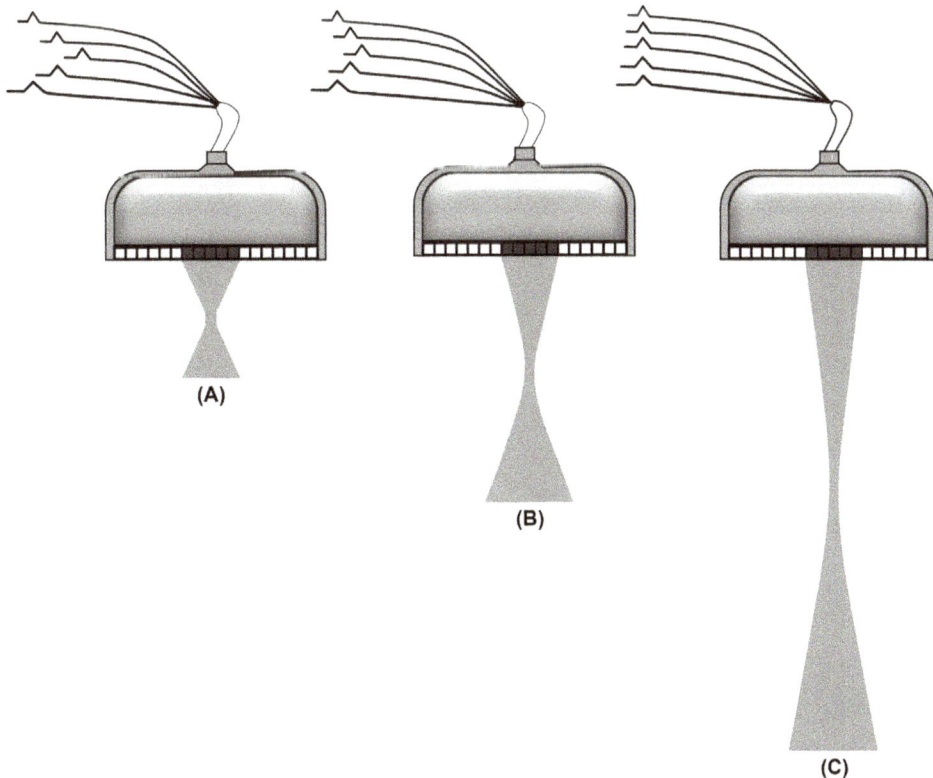

FIGURE 3-12. Focal length for a crystal group is varied by changing the timed-excitation pulses to the crystals, depending on the degree of focusing desired. **(A)** Short focus. **(B)** Medium focus. **(C)** Long focus.

Most traditional scanners allow the operator to select the number and location of focal zones (although only one focal zone may be permitted in combined modes or for application presets where the maximum frame rate is required, such as cardiac). However, some point-of-care systems automatically set the number and location of focal zones based on the examination type (preset) and the display depth selected.

Aperture Focusing

Electronic focusing during transmission also involves varying the number of crystals activated in the segment to alter the size of the radiating surface or aperture (Figure 3-13). The aperture is increased to maintain relatively narrow beam width for longer focal lengths. For example, two crystals are fired as a group to produce a very short, narrow field near the transducer. If more crystals are added in the group, then the depth before rapid divergence is extended, but the beam width near the transducer is broadened

(dictated by the radiating surface). Large aperture improves focusing at extended depths. Manufacturers employ combinations of time-delayed firing and changing beam aperture to optimize focusing at different depths. The focal zone is the region over which the beam width is most narrow and the depth of field (length of the focal zone) for a multiple-element array depends on aperture, focal length, and frequency.

Apodization

Apodization employs a variable-strength voltage pulse to the crystals across the aperture during transmit focusing. The excitation voltage to the individual crystals in each group is maximized at the center and reduced toward the periphery (Figure 3-14). This technique reduces the intensity of side lobes (sound radiating in directions different from the main beam) in multiple-element arrays. High frequency and large number of similar elements in the active area of an

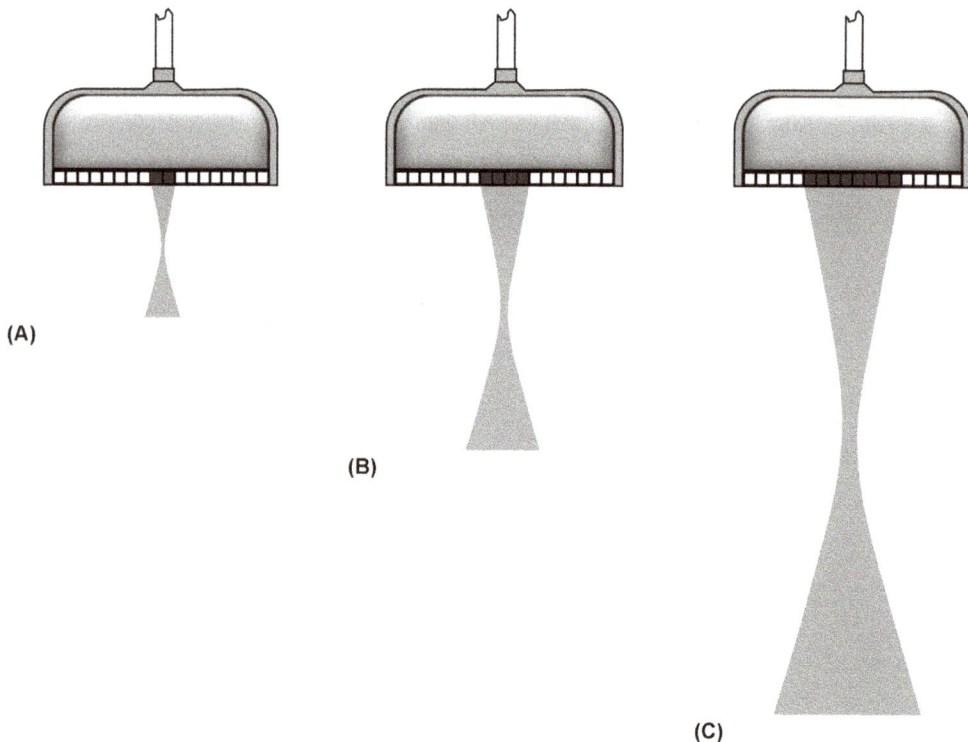

(A)

(B)

(C)

FIGURE 3-13. Aperture focusing. Two crystals are fired for short focus **(A)**, four crystals for medium focus **(B)**, and eight crystals for long focus **(C)**.

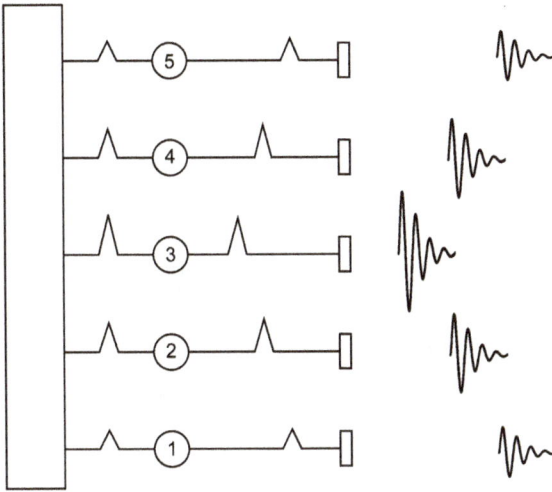

FIGURE 3-14. Apodization varies the strength of the voltage pulse to each crystal (represented by different peak heights in a five-crystal segment) to improve focusing. The highest voltage is applied to the center crystal which generates the most dominant waveform.

array (effectively creating a larger radiating surface) reduce the intensity of side lobes.

Digital Beam Former

Beam management during transmission (scanning and focusing) for multiple-element arrays is performed by a digital beam former. The complex combination of time delays, aperture, and apodization are most effectively applied with digital electronics during transmission. Compared with analog devices, digital beam formers allow greater flexibility in beam manipulation with regard to ultrasonic field shape, beam width, direction, and intensity.

DYNAMIC RECEIVE FOCUSING

Another means to reduce the effective sampling volume is dynamic focusing in the receive mode. In essence, the echo-induced signals across several elements are combined to enhance the overall signal originating from a single reflector. The following analogy illustrates the principle of receive focus. Three runners of equal ability begin a race at the same starting point but follow

different routes to the finish line. At the finish line, an observer is assigned to each runner and must shout the point of origin when the runner crosses the finish line. Because the distance traveled by each runner is not identical, three separate shouts are heard as the race is completed. If an obstacle, such as a wall, is placed in the path of each runner, the sequence of finish can be regulated. The height of the wall is adjusted depending on the distance between the starting point and the finish line. To increase the delay before crossing the finish line, the height of the obstacle is made greater. In this case, the shortest route would incorporate the tallest wall. For a certain combination of obstacles, the runners finish the race simultaneously, and one loud shout is heard from all the observers identifying the point of origin. The race can be made more complex by varying the starting point. The heights of the obstacles can be adjusted according to the change in distance. Now the observers are given a chart that denotes the starting point based on the elapsed time of the race. This is possible because the participants run at the same speed. The shouts of the observers at the finish line are still synchronized; only the words to identify the starting points vary. Dynamic receive focusing works in a similar manner.

By means of time-delay circuitry in the receiver, the induced signals from the returning ultrasound wave are refocused when multiple crystals receive the echo. Dynamic focusing is not limited to one fixed depth per transmitted pulse, as transmit focusing is, but is applied continuously for all depths. In Figure 3-15, five crystals receive the echo reflected toward the transducer from the object. The ultrasound beam diverges during its return to the transducer and strikes the five crystals at different times. The wavefront intercepts crystal 3 first, then crystals 2 and 4, and finally crystals 1 and 5. By using receiver time delays, the echo-induced signal at crystal 3 is delayed until the wavefront reaches crystals 1 and 5. Similarly, the echo-induced signals from crystals 2 and 4 are delayed until the wavefront reaches crystals 1 and 5, although the delay time is shorter than that for crystal 3. The actual time delay is determined for each crystal by simple geometry and an assumed constant acoustic velocity in

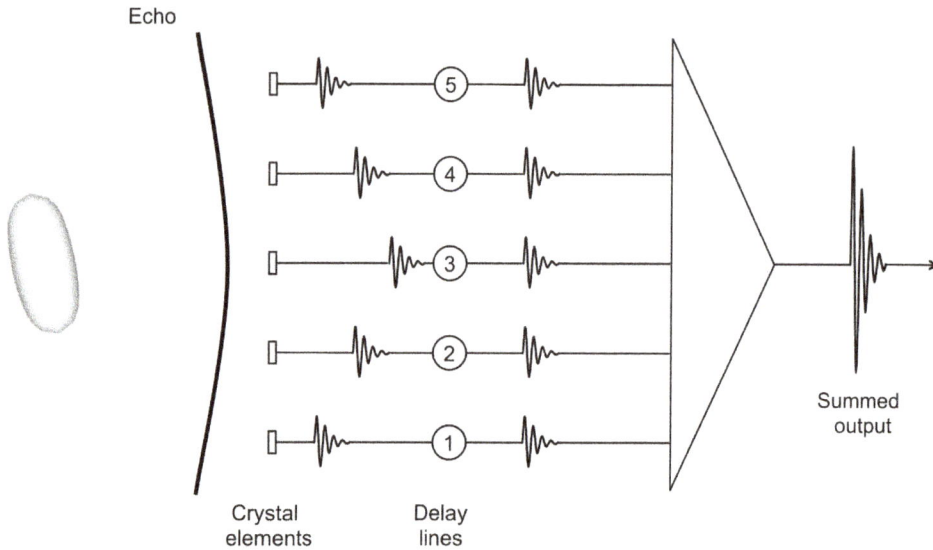

FIGURE 3-15. Dynamic receive focusing. The echo wavefront from the reflector does not reach all crystals in the array at the same time. By delaying the individual echo-induced signal at each crystal until the wavefront has arrived at all five crystals, focusing is applied to the received signals to produce a summed output.

soft tissue. The wavefront from the reflector appears to be in phase for all five crystals, resulting in a "focused" beam from that depth of sampling. This delay and sum strategy is called receive beam formation.

The same principle applies to the echo-induced signals arising from a reflector located farther from the transducer. Because of the greater depth, the wavefront strikes the crystals with less variability and a shorter series of receiver time delays focuses the detected signals from the reflector. The elapsed time from transmission to reception determines the delay time for each crystal within the group. The depth for receive focus is always known, and thus receiver time delays are continually changed to yield a receive-focused beam at all depths. That is, during acquisition of scan data, the receiver time delays are varied dynamically to sweep the received focal zone to each point along the scan line.

The received beam width is uniformly narrow along the scan line. In essence, therefore, spatial registration is improved by restricting the tissue volume that contributes to each pixel along the scan line. A dynamic receive aperture adjusts the number of active crystals during reception to optimize focusing as a

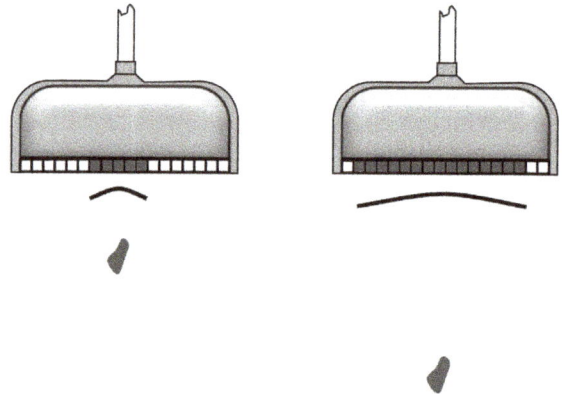

FIGURE 3-16. Receive aperture. The number of elements that compose the received signal increases with depth.

function of depth. Additional elements are included in the aperture as the depth of the focal zone is increased (Figure 3-16). *Dynamic receive focusing is achieved without a loss in frame rate or line density.*

Dynamic receive focusing is improved as the number of crystals forming the summed signal is increased. Compare the spatial resolution at a depth of 8 cm for the sonograms obtained with 64 versus 128 receive channels (Figure 3-17).

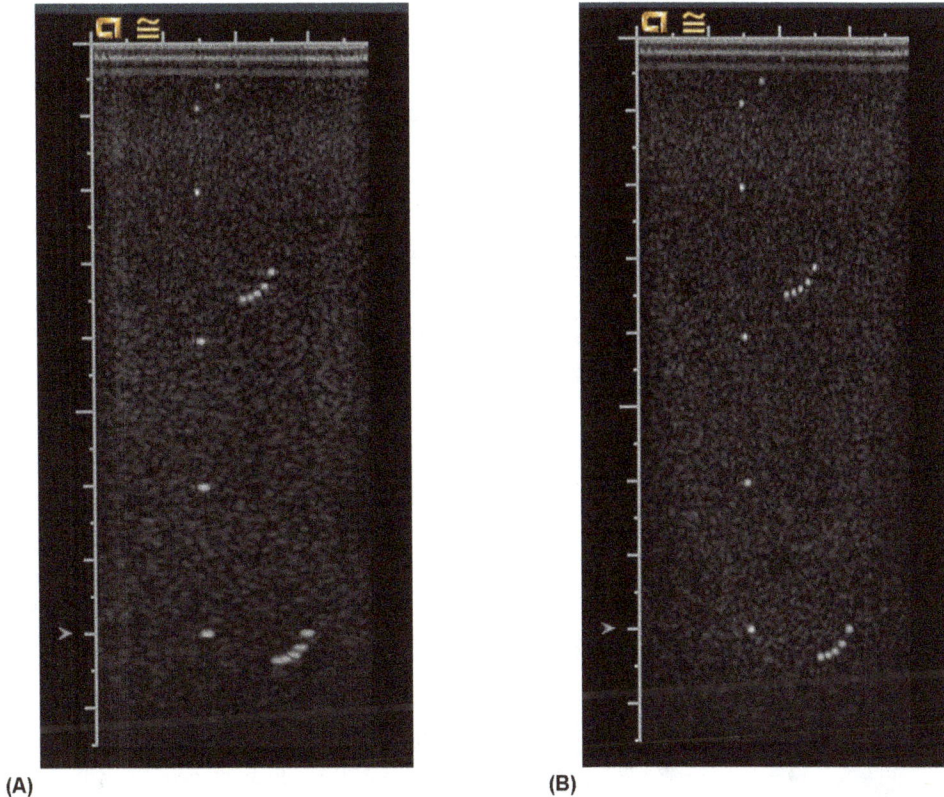

FIGURE 3-17. Effect of channel number. Sonograms of a tissue-mimicking phantom with 64 receive channels **(A)** and 128 receive channels **(B)**. Note the improved spatial detail as channel number is increased. (Courtesy Rob Steins.)

CURVILINEAR ARRAY

In the past few years, the curvilinear (also called convex or curved) array that portrays a large trapezoid-shaped field of view has been developed. The curvilinear array contains 128–256 crystal elements arranged along an arc in a linear, sequential fashion. The radius of curvature is usually 25–100 mm. A large radius of curvature expands the width of the field of view. Unlike a linear array, the width of the field of view is not restricted to the physical length of the assembled crystals. Similar to linear arrays, the physical dimensions of the crystal elements, the number of elements excited, and the timing sequence influence the beam pattern.

Curvilinear arrays sweep the beam by select activation of multiple crystals in a group, and after the appropriate delay transmission is offset to the next group. The curved crystal arrangement provides scan lines that are perpendicular to the array surface (Figure 3-18). Scan lines are not parallel to one another, but radiate outward in different directions due to the curved geometry of the transducer face (Figure 3-19). Scan line density is decreased at depth and a loss of spatial definition can occur. In-plane transmit focusing and mechanical focusing in the elevation direction, similar to the linear array, are also applied.

PHASED ARRAY

Another electronic, multiple-element transducer, the phased array, was developed to overcome certain limitations inherent in the linear array, most notably the large size of the linear array footprint. The phased array is now commonly referred to as simply sector,

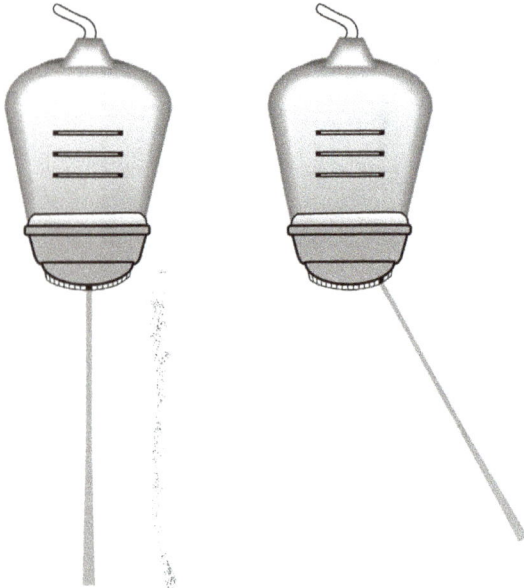

FIGURE 3-18. Curvilinear array. Control of scan line direction is by element selection. Two scan lines are shown.

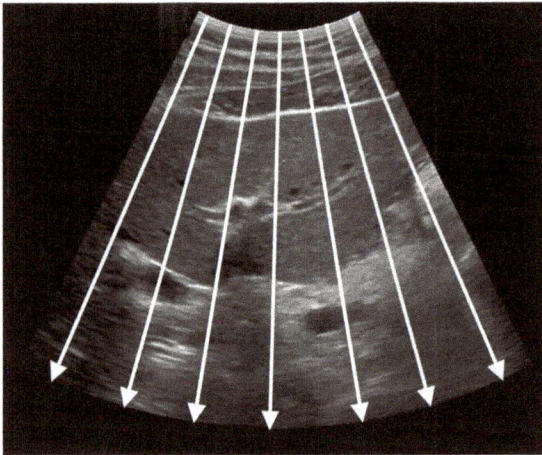

FIGURE 3-19. The direction and orientation of scan lines shown for an image obtained with a curvilinear array transducer.

which has its origin in the image format produced by this type of transducer. Image formation with a linear array produces a rectangular field of view in which the width is determined by the physical length of the row of elements and the maximum number of scan lines is limited by the number of elements in the array. The relatively low number of scan lines

per frame allows high frame rates, but spatial detail is sacrificed. The large footprint of the linear array (several centimeters in length) prevents access to structures where a narrow acoustic window is available (e.g., between the ribs for cardiac imaging).

Phased arrays contain multiple, rectangular crystals of approximately 100 elements arranged side by side in a straight row with a small footprint. To generate and direct the ultrasonic beam, all (or most) of the crystals in the phased array are excited nearly simultaneously. This contrasts with linear arrays, in which the crystals are stimulated in small groups. The phased array produces a sector format with a sector angle as large as 90 degrees. Scan lines diverge with depth and therefore, scan line density is not constant throughout the field of view. Restricting the field of view with a small sector angle (e.g., 30 degrees) allows high frame rate and/or increased scan line density. For example, an image composed of 150 scan lines can be updated 30 times per second if the scan range is 15 cm. Phased arrays are commonly employed in echocardiology, because their small size (10–30 mm in length) enables better access to the heart through small acoustic windows.

Electronic steering of the beam across the field of view allows data collection along different scan lines. The entire phased array produces a single scan line each time the array of crystal elements is excited. Beam direction is controlled by the timing sequence of the voltage stimulation to the individual crystal elements. When excited each crystal produces a circular wavefront, which moves into tissue. Since the origins of the individual wavefronts from the various elements are shifted with respect to location and time, they add together to create a resultant wave. By altering the timing order of the excitation pulses across the array, the direction of propagation of the transmitted beam can be varied to any desired scan angle (Figure 3-20). The scan angle is denoted as the angle between the direction of propagation and the normal to the central element in the array. The composite of multiple scan lines oriented at different scan angles forms the sector image (Figure 3-21). For phased arrays the number of scan lines is not limited by the number of elements in the array.

Additional small time adjustments are applied for transmit-focusing purposes as the beam is steered. As

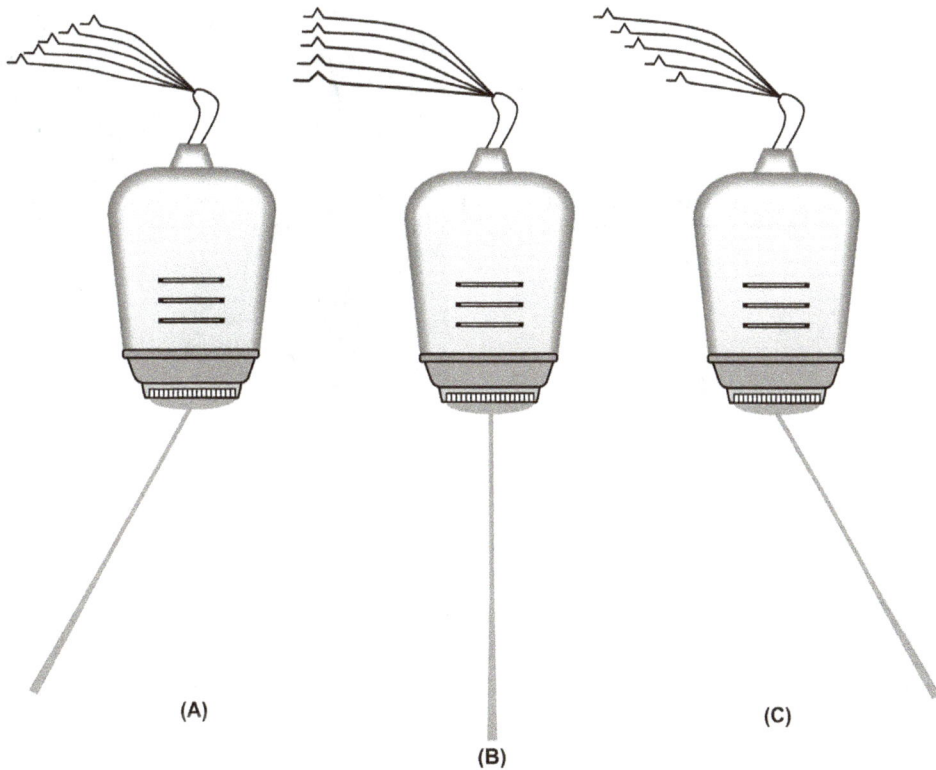

FIGURE 3-20. Beam steering with a phased array. (**A** through **C**) The excitation timing sequence for the crystals in the array is changed to steer the beam in different directions. For illustration purposes only five channels are shown, but 100 channels are common.

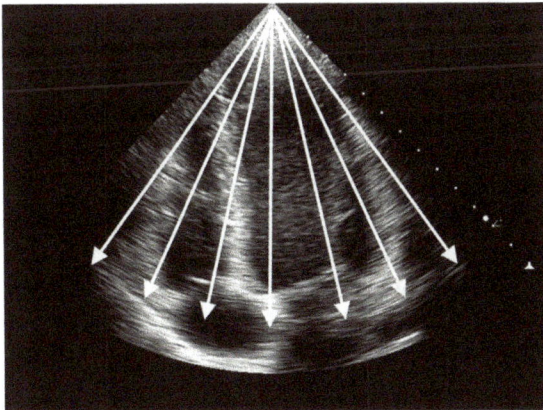

FIGURE 3-21. The direction and orientation of scan lines shown for an image obtained with a phased array transducer.

with other multiple-element arrays, transmit focusing is limited to one focal point for each transmitted beam. Once data have been collected along this scan line, the focal point can be changed (by modifying the delay line timing) to rescan this scan line with a new focal length. In this manner, the transmit focal zone can be positioned at different depths. This reduces the in-plane beam width within the focal zone. However, multiple zone transmit focusing slows the frame rate, because multiple transmit pulses are necessary to compose each scan line. The phased array can also be dynamically focused in the receive mode. Outside the central field of view, spatial resolution deteriorates, because electronic focusing becomes more difficult when large-angle beam steering is performed. Phased arrays are mechanically focused in the elevation (slice thickness) direction.

STEERED LINEAR ARRAY

The principle of electronic steering as with a phased array can also be applied to the linear array to form a scanned field of view, which is oriented at an

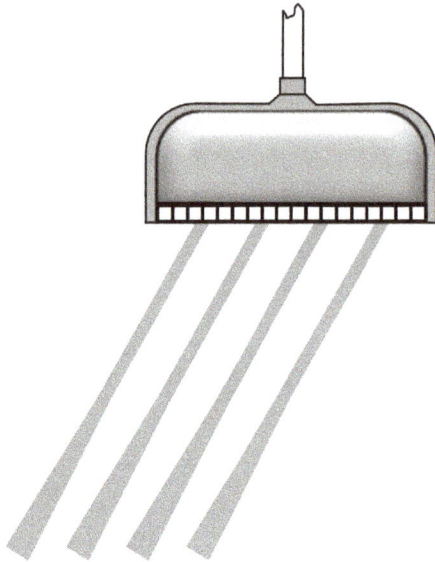

FIGURE 3-22. Steered linear array. Electronic steering directs the scan lines at an angle relative to the radiating surface. The scan lines are parallel at the same respective angle to the array.

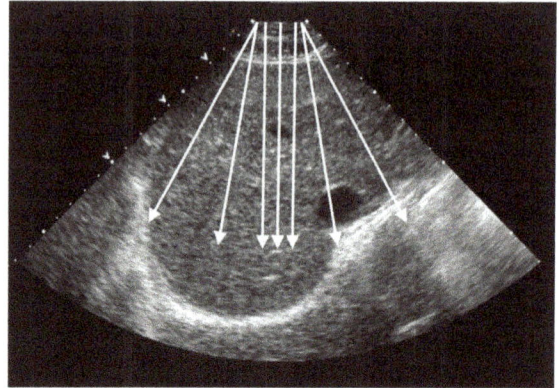

FIGURE 3-23. The direction and orientation of scan lines shown for an image obtained with a vector array transducer.

angle to the crystal row. This type of transducer is called a steered linear array. The B-mode image is composed of parallel scan lines, each directed at the same angle from the array (Figure 3-22). Analogous to the linear array, the number of scan lines is limited by the number of elements in the array. By steering the beam, the most favorable angle of interrogation can be selected for the reflector of interest. This technique is also commonly used in color Doppler imaging.

VECTOR ARRAY

The vector array (also called compound linear and virtual convex) incorporates characteristics from both the linear array and the phased array. In fact, this transducer is classified as a phased array by some manufacturers. Scan lines for the central field of view are obtained by selective excitation of elements so that the beam path is perpendicular to the array (same as the linear array). At the extremes of the field of view, the ultrasound beam is steered at wide angles by the phased method. An enlarged effective field of view that extends beyond the physical length of the array is created (Figure 3-23). In-plane transmit focusing and mechanical focusing in the elevation direction, similar to the other multiple-element arrays, are also applied. The footprint is smaller than that for the curvilinear array, and the field of view is trapezoidal in shape with a small, flat border near the transducer face.

1.5D ARRAY

A major weakness of the previously described multiple-element arrays is the inability to apply dynamic focusing to control the slice thickness of the transmitted beam. Focusing in the elevation plane is commonly accomplished by an acoustic lens with a fixed focal length. Within the mechanical focal zone the slice thickness is 3–5 mm, but outside the focal zone slice thickness can increase significantly. Compare this to an in-plane beam width of about 1 mm, which is achievable by electronic focusing. This relatively large elevation beam width creates partial volume artifacts when imaging small structures. Contours may be blurred because the detected signal is a combination of the small reflector and the surrounding tissue. The 1.5D array transducer provides electronic focusing in the elevation plane.

The single row of elements in the conventional linear array is replaced by three to seven rows of smaller elements in the 1.5D array (Figure 3-24). Beam direction is determined by element selection.

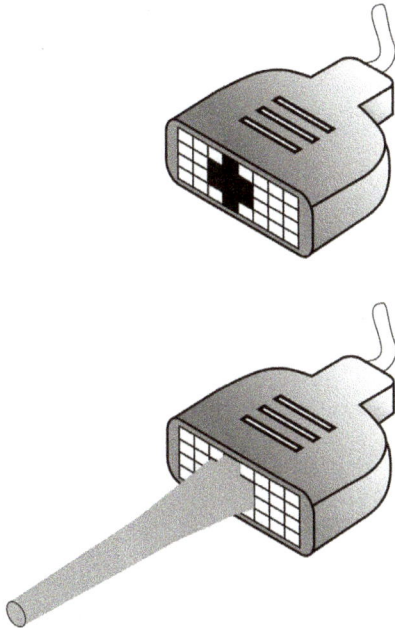

FIGURE 3-24. 1.5D transducer. By subdividing each crystal in a linear array to form multiple rows of crystals, variable focusing in the elevation direction is possible. The location of the focal zone depends on element selection (shown in black, above) and the timing sequence.

The additional crystal elements in the adjacent rows are activated with time delay channels to enable electronic focusing in the elevation plane.

TRANSDUCER COMPARISON

Characteristics of the six ultrasound transducers introduced in this chapter are summarized in Table 3-1. Selection of the optimal transducer for a particular clinical application depends on these properties, such as footprint and image format. An important additional consideration is the operating frequency. Clinical applications are discussed in Chapter 7.

TRANSDUCER CARE

A transducer is susceptible to damage if dropped or sustains an impact. A cracked transducer surface is potentially dangerous to the operator and the patient, and must be removed from service. The repeated twisting and bending of the cable can lead to transducer malfunction. During transport, care must

TABLE 3-1 • Transducer Characteristics

Type	Scanning Mechanism	In-Plane Focusing	Elevation Focusing	Image Format	Footprint
Linear array	Electronic sequencing	Electronic	Mechanical	Rectangular	Flat
Curvilinear array	Electronic sequencing	Electronic	Mechanical	Trapezoidal	Curved
Phased array	Electronic steering	Electronic	Mechanical	Sector	Flat
Steered array	Electronic sequencing and steering	Electronic	Mechanical	Skewed rectangle	Flat
Vector array	Electronic sequencing and steering	Electronic	Mechanical	Trapezoidal	Flat
1.5D array	Electronic sequencing	Electronic	Electronic	Rectangular	Flat

be taken to prevent damage to the transducers and cables.

Many transducers are not watertight, and thus immersion in liquids can damage the transducer. The preferred cleaning method is a damp cloth moistened with soap and water. If decontamination of bodily fluids is required, then disinfecting and sterilizing solutions usually containing glutaraldehyde are used. Intracavitary probes are soaked *for a prescribed time* in the disinfecting liquid. Extended immersion in the liquid can damage the intracavitary probe. *The manufacturer's recommendations for cleaning should be followed exactly.*

Gas sterilization, ultraviolet sterilization, dry heat sterilization, autoclaving, and soaking in chlorine bleach can damage the transducer and must be avoided. If sterility is required, then the transducer is placed in a sterile sleeve with sterile coupling gel applied to the interior and exterior near the transducer face.

Chemical agents containing acetone, mineral oil, iodine, and oil-based perfume can also damage the transducer. Coupling gels with these chemical agents should not be used. The manufacturer usually provides a listing of approved products.

References

Hangiandreous NJ: B-mode US: basic concepts and new technology. Radiographics 23, 1019–1033, 2003.

Hedrick WR: Technology for diagnostic sonography, St. Louis, 2013, Elsevier.

Hedrick WR, Hykes DL: Beam steering and focusing with linear phased arrays. Journal of Diagnostic Medical Sonography 12, 211–215, 1996.

Hedrick WR, Hykes DL, Starchman DE: Ultrasound physics and instrumentation, ed 4, St. Louis, 2005, Elsevier.

Hykes DL, Hedrick WR: Real-time ultrasound instrumentation. Journal of Diagnostic Medical Sonography 6, 257–268, 1990.

Kremkau FW: Multiple-element transducers. Radiographics 13, 1163–1176, 1993.

Kremkau FW: Diagnostic ultrasound: principles and instruments, ed 8, Philadelphia, 2011, WB Saunders.

Zagzebski JA: Essentials of ultrasound physics, St Louis, 1996, Mosby-Year Book.

4

Real-Time B-Mode Imaging

OBJECTIVES

- To be familiar with B-mode operator controls.

- To understand the various operational modes of real-time B-mode imaging.

KEY TERMS

3D imaging

4D ultrasound

Cine

Display depth

Dual display

Dynamic range

Elastography

Extended field of view

Frame averaging

Freeze

Gain

Gray-scale mapping

M-mode

Optimize

Output power

Reject

Sector width

Spatial compounding

Temporal resolution

Time gain compensation (TGC)

Tissue harmonic imaging

Transmit focus

Transmit frequency

Zoom

OPERATOR CONTROLS

Ultrasound scanners are very sophisticated devices that require operator interaction to obtain accurate diagnostic information. No other imaging modality is more dependent on operator input during image acquisition as well as processing for optimal image quality. An array of operator controls has been developed to enhance the scanning process, although devices vary in the types of controls that are available (Figure 4-1). Within each examination type, proper control settings vary from patient to patient based on age, size, weight,

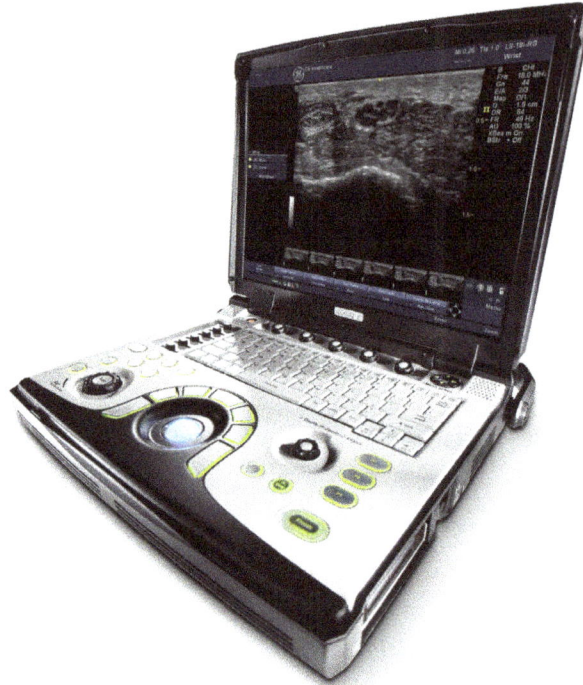

(A)

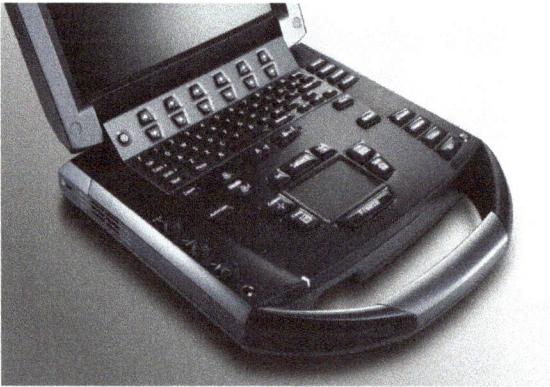

(B)

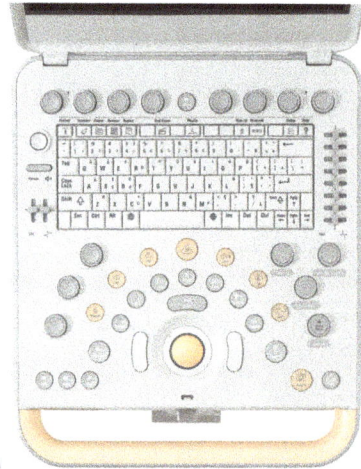

(C)

FIGURE 4-1. Operator control panel for three scanners (A) GE Logiq-e (Courtesy of GE Healthcare), (B) Sonosite Edge (Courtesy of FujiFILM-Sonosite, Inc.), (C) (Courtesy of Philips Healthcare).

body habitus, and disease process. For a single sonographic examination of the abdomen, scanning may include the liver, kidneys, gallbladder, and great vessels. Transmit focus, display depth, gain, and transmit frequency must be adjusted repeatedly to obtain the best possible images. Indeed, the time gain compensation control must be verified or adjusted when the transducer is oriented to a new imaging plane.

Traditionally, the entire complement of operator controls was available on every ultrasound instrument, although the name and style of some controls (knobs, switches, trackball, etc.) varied according to the manufacturer. Transducer and examination presets were programmed to specific default values determined to be optimal for the selected examination type. From the initial starting configuration, the user could manually adjust most parameters to further optimize the image while maintaining desired output power settings. Point-of-care instruments present a distinct deviation from this well-accepted practice. Although all of these controls still exist in some form on the system, many are not readily accessible by the operator. Instruments from several manufacturers exhibit a wide variation in console design and extent of user control. Some instruments permit direct operator adjustment of most, if not all, traditional parameters, while other manufacturers have adopted a completely different approach. In these streamlined systems, parameters such as time gain compensation, depth and number of focal zones, frame rate, and output power are automatically assigned according to the examination type, display depth, and transducer selected by the operator. Analysis of returning echoes enables further refinement of parameter settings, which are also transparent to the operator. Therefore, the sonographer must select the correct exam preset, display depth, and overall gain, since appropriate settings for these parameters are essential to ensure optimal values for focus, transmit frequency, output power, and other acquisition parameters not directly accessible to the user.

Transmit Frequency

Transducers are designed to operate at a single center frequency or over a wide range of variable frequencies during transmission and reception (designated as broadband transducers). In the latter circumstance, the desirable transmit frequency is selected within the possible range and then may be altered during scanning without physically switching to a different transducer. Other terms for transmit frequency include operating frequency, center frequency, and

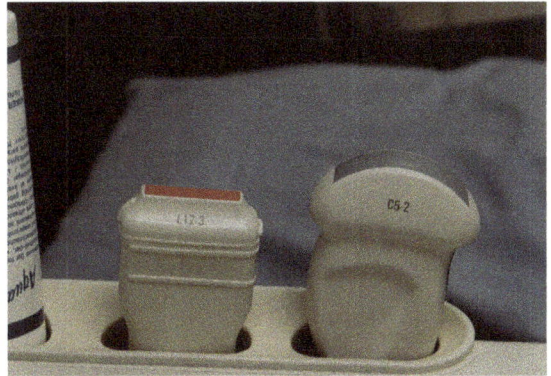

FIGURE 4-2. Broadband linear array transducer with an operating range of 3–12 MHz and broadband curvilinear array transducer with an operating range of 2–5 MHz.

nominal frequency. Transducers are typically labeled to denote the frequency range within which the given transducer functions, as shown in Figure 4-2. In this example, the label "L12-3" refers to a linear array transducer with a frequency range of 3-12 MHz. Some manufacturers utilize a single frequency to denote the midpoint of the frequency range, while other manufacturers specify the maximum frequency only.

The first and most obvious way to set the transmit frequency is by the choice of the transducer most appropriate for the exam. Transducer selection is based on the examination to be performed, which includes transducer design (sector, linear, curvilinear, or endocavitary) and suitable frequency range. For example, an adult echocardiogram would dictate the choice of a sector transducer. However, the operator may have the choice between two different phased array transducers, one with a range of 2.25–3.5 MHz and another with a range of 3.5–5.0 MHz. The highest frequency that allows penetration to the anatomy of interest should be selected, since spatial resolution is improved as frequency is increased.

Manufacturers have controls that enable the operator to adjust the transmit frequency up or down, but the terminology is often vendor-specific. Labels for the frequency selection control include "frequency fusion," "multihertz," and "transmit frequency." Incremental increases and decreases in the frequency control may be shown on the display as a specific

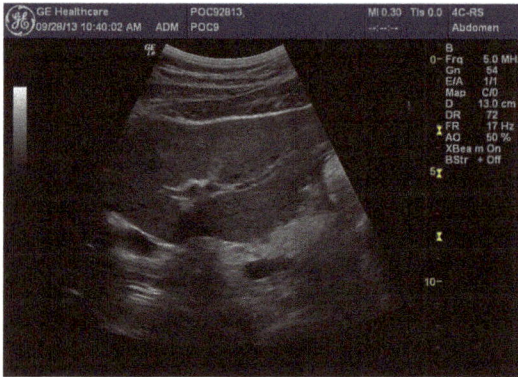

FIGURE 4-3. Abdominal sonogram obtained at 5 MHz with a scan range of 13 cm.

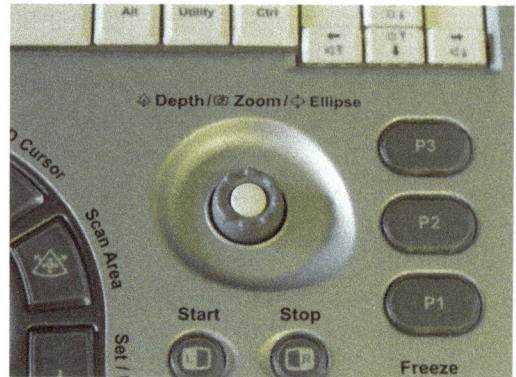

FIGURE 4-5. Display depth (scan range) control.

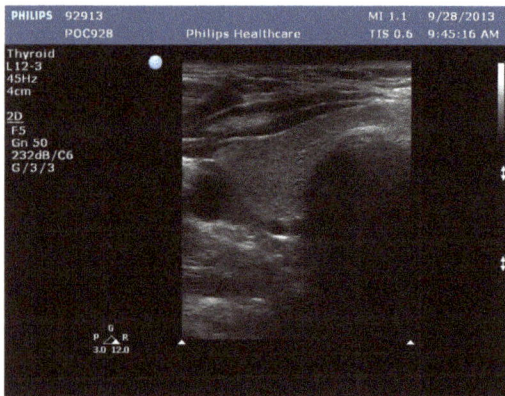

FIGURE 4-4. Thyroid sonogram obtained at 15 MHz with a scan range of 4 cm.

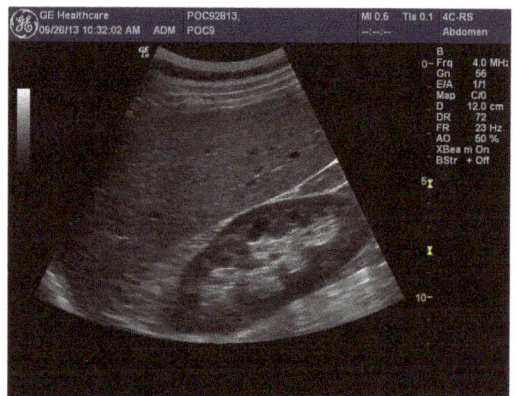

FIGURE 4-6. Sonogram of the liver and right kidney with a scan range of 12 cm.

value such as "5 MHz," or may simply be indicated as "R" for "resolution" and as "P" for "penetration." To obtain the best spatial resolution, scanning should be performed at the highest practical frequency, while still maintaining adequate penetration to image the organ of interest (Figures 4-3 and 4-4).

Display Depth

Display depth control adjusts the scan range to best represent the anatomy of interest (Figure 4-5). Generally, the depth of the field of view should be set one to a few centimeters beyond the deepest part of the scanned organ (Figure 4-6). The real-time frame rate may be reduced as scan range is extended, since more

time is required for the ultrasound pulse to travel to and the echo to return from the maximum depth (time of flight). As a consequence, the transducer transmits fewer pulses in a given time period and the time to complete one frame (one complete set of scan lines across the field of view) is longer. Increased time to compose a frame lowers the maximum frame rate. In conjunction with a change in display depth, manufacturers often automatically adjust the pulse repetition frequency or scan line density to maintain a constant frame rate. Some manufacturers link other parameters to display depth, such as number and location of focal zones, transmit/receive frequency, and output power.

Freeze Frame, Cine

The freeze control enables the operator to review still images and real-time video clips (Figure 4-7). Scan data acquisition is discontinued while the freeze-frame option is selected. The most recently acquired frames can then be recalled from the system memory (typically 100–200 frames). Activation of the review function is usually done simply by scrolling the trackball backward or using the left and right arrows to view stored images frame by frame (Figure 4-8). The most recently acquired images held in the buffer can also be viewed in temporal sequence by activating the cine function (retrospective mode). On some systems, the cine function can be operated in a prospective mode in which images are captured immediately after this control is turned on.

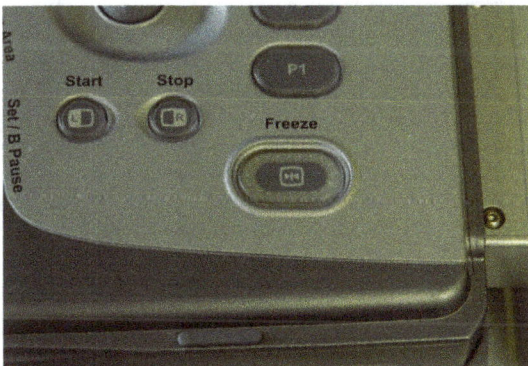

FIGURE 4-7. Freeze control.

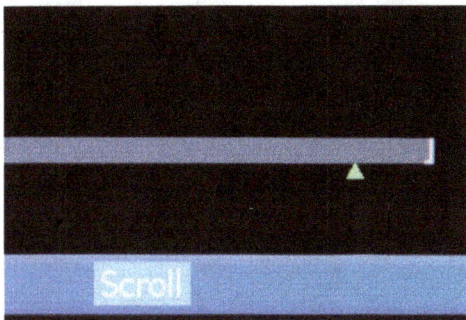

FIGURE 4-8. Frame selection during image review.

Images captured in the buffer are not permanently stored and will be lost during subsequent scan/freeze cycles. Reviewed images and video clips can be transferred to internal storage (hard disk) for record keeping purposes using image save or cine save.

Correct "freeze" operation requires extensive clinical experience. During live scanning, the operator's non-transducer hand should be on or near the freeze button. Proficiency in freezing the image requires proper timing with patient respiration and organ movement. Although the ability to scroll backward through stored frames can result in a useable image for a difficult patient, this practice should be avoided as a substitute for good freeze technique. Activating the review function routinely on every stored image extends examination time and may not result in optimal image quality.

Gain

During signal processing, **receiver gain, overall gain**, or gain amplifies the echo-induced signals equally throughout the scan range and is often expressed in decibels or in percentage. The amount of amplification is quantified as the ratio of the output signal to the input signal. Noise and signal are increased by the same relative amount and thus, the signal-to-noise ratio and the depth of penetration are unchanged by adjusting the gain control. Consequently, gain is manipulated to establish the proper brightness level for image display (Figure 4-9), but it generally does not improve the detection of weak reflectors. Within certain limitations (weak signals are not enhanced), the visual effect of increased gain is the same as increased output power. The gain control, unlike the power control, does not affect the rate at which ultrasound energy is delivered into the patient.

Auto gain automatically sets the brightness of the image each time the key is pressed. The overall brightness is sensed by weighing the respective gray levels of all the pixels. This control is useful to establish the initial gain setting, which can then be modified as appropriate with manual adjustment of the gain control.

(A)

(B)

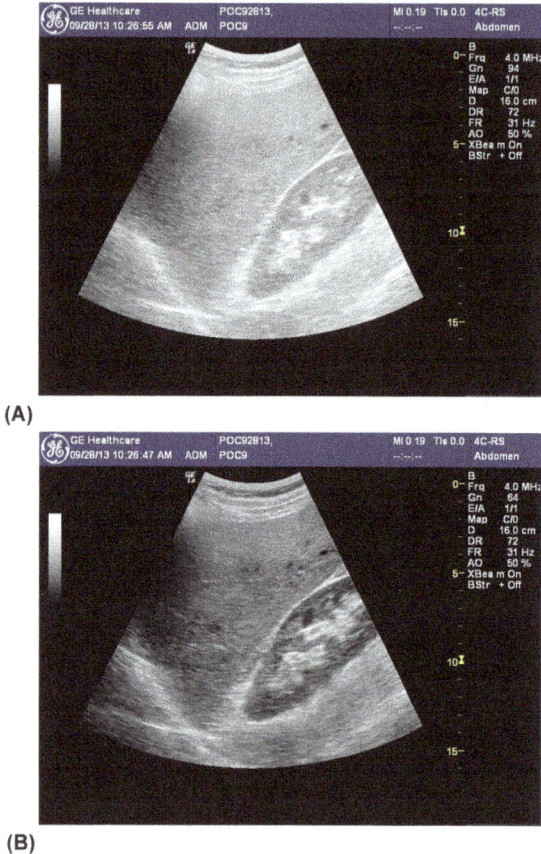

FIGURE 4-9. Image quality comparison showing the effect of gain. (**A**) Gain set too high. (**B**) Proper gain setting.

Output Power

The output power control varies the excitation voltage applied to the transducer elements (Figure 4-10). Power levels are commonly expressed in decibels or

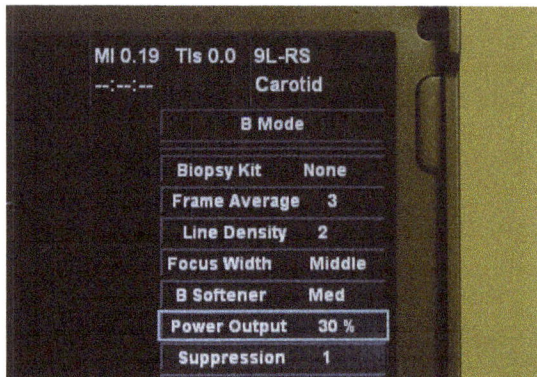

FIGURE 4-10. Transmit power set at 30%.

percentage (e.g., 0 dB or 100% indicates full power and −3 dB or 50% corresponds to half maximum power). The excitation voltage governs the intensity of the sound transmitted into the patient and, subsequently, the strength of the echo from a reflector. A high-power setting improves the system sensitivity to detect weak reflectors and extends the depth of penetration (Figure 4-11), but also causes increased image brightness. The visual effect on the B-mode image is similar to an adjustment of the overall gain. Some systems automatically adjust the gain in conjunction with an altered power setting to maintain overall image brightness at a constant level.

Obtaining the appropriate image brightness is a balance between output power and receiver gain settings. The ability to adjust image brightness to the

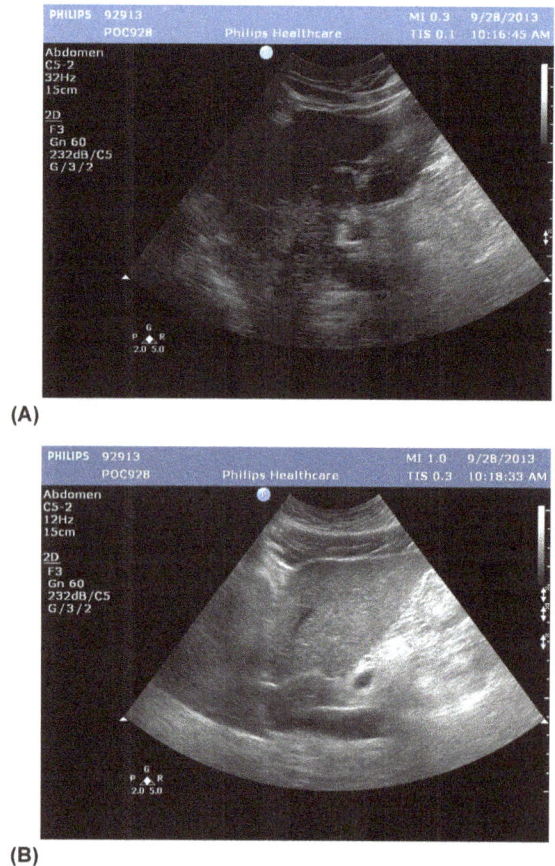

(A)

(B)

FIGURE 4-11. Visualization of weak reflectors is improved with increased power. (**A**) Transmit power set too low and (**B**) Adequate output power setting.

optimal level with the gain control depends upon an adequate power setting. Ideally, the system should be set at the minimum output power necessary to image the structure/depth of interest. Additional image brightness is achieved by increasing the gain.

The following guideline is recommended for the proper adjustment of gain and output power. If more image brightness is required, *first* increase the overall gain. If that does not result in adequate image brightness, then increase the output power. If less image brightness is required, *first* decrease the output power. If that is not sufficient to produce the correct image brightness, then decrease the overall gain. By observing this guideline, the operator is applying the principle of ALARA and the patient is exposed to the lowest ultrasound energy.

Time Gain Compensation (TGC)

Attenuation causes the sound wave to lose energy as it travels through tissue. Echoes that originate from extended depths are considerably weakened by attenuation. Time gain compensation (TGC) is a type of receiver gain that is varied according to time (depth) to correct for attenuation along the beam path. Without compensation for attenuation, an echo originating from a deep-lying reflector would appear less bright (darker shade of gray) than an echo created from that same reflector at a more shallow depth. Ideally, structures with identical reflectivity appear as the same shade of gray on the display unrelated to depth. Time gain compensation is applied automatically to amplify echo-induced signals conditionally based on the depth of formation (time delay after the transmitted pulsed wave) and is dependent on the display depth setting and the examination preset selected. Some point-of-care systems, particularly the smaller hand-held models, do not allow user adjustment of TGC. Instead they rely solely on display depth setting and examination presets. Thus, the application preset and display depth must be correct.

Fine adjustment of TGC, when operator controlled, utilizes a set of sliders or keys for near gain and far gain (Figure 4-12). Near gain adjusts the gain in the region near the transducer and far gain

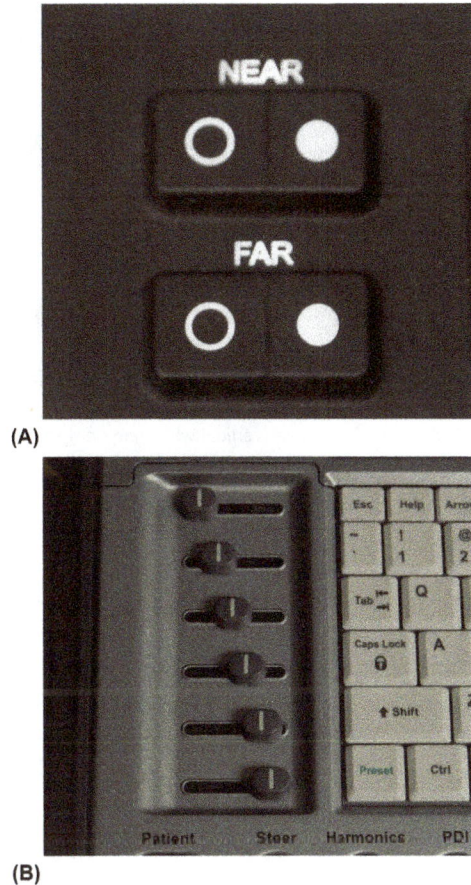

(A)

(B)

FIGURE 4-12. Controls for time gain compensation. (**A**) Keys. (**B**) Sliders.

adjusts the gain at the limits of the scan range. Use of multiple sliders provides the capability to make adjustments to the TGC. Each slider on the TGC panel corresponds to a specific depth and simultaneously a specific region on the screen associated with that depth. Each slider may be individually adjusted as necessary to apply the appropriate amplification so that a uniformly bright image is produced. TGC slider placements are adjusted based on visual appearance of the image, rather than by specific numeric values.

The respective positions of the TGC sliders produce a profile of amplification called a gain curve, which is a graph of the variable gain as a function of time/depth. This gain curve is often displayed next to the two-dimensional (2D) image so that points along the time/depth axis correspond visually to the image

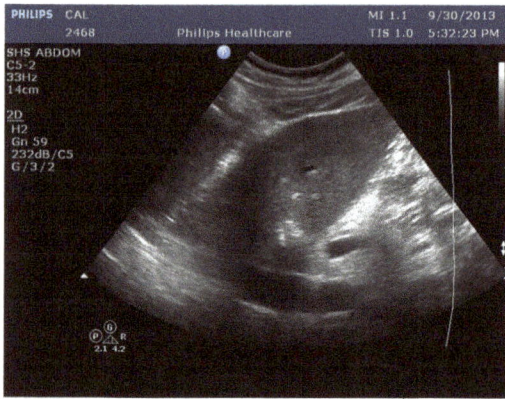

FIGURE 4-13. Gain curve (vertical white line on right side of image).

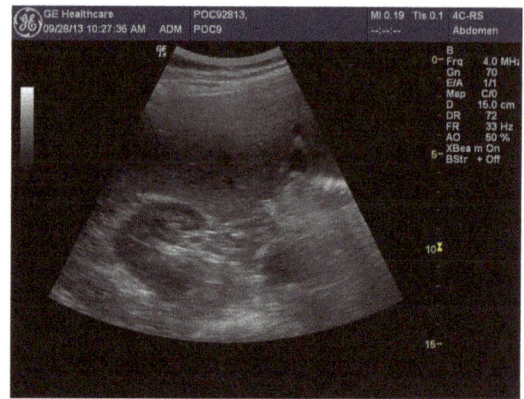

FIGURE 4-14. Improper TGC adjustment. Note the dark banding effect seen across the image at approximately 5 cm depth on the display.

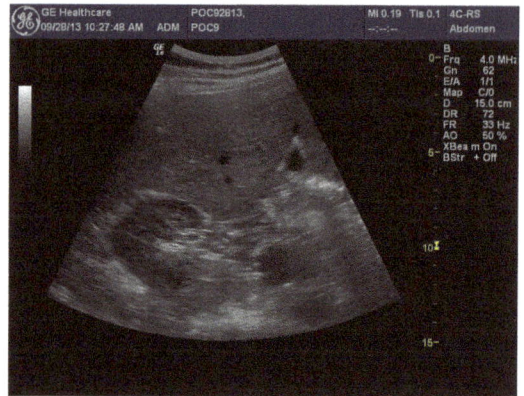

FIGURE 4-15. Correct adjustment of TGC.

(Figure 4-13). The gain curve may also be envisioned by observing the relative slider positions at different depths, as shown in Figure 4-12B.

A straight-line gain curve is generally appropriate only for a homogeneous medium, which is not representative of the human body. A sound wave transmitted from the transducer into the body must first pass through the abdominal or chest wall composed of muscle, fat, and connective tissue prior to reaching the organ(s) of interest, such as the liver or the heart. The imaged organs may have heterogeneous as well as homogeneous regions, including fluid-filled structures such as blood vessels, heart chambers, or urinary bladder.

Tissue along the propagation path attenuates sound at different rates and therefore, a uniquely adjusted TGC curve is required for each scan plane. In addition, signal-generating sources often occur immediately beyond the transducer face and within the extreme far field. The TGC control can be utilized to minimize the effect of these distracting signals in the display.

In practice, a "standard" TGC curve based on exam type takes into account the above issues. This results in a nonlinear curve that emphasizes or de-emphasizes certain sections of the image. An improperly adjusted TGC may cause dark or white banding (unsuitable low or high gain) and reduced information content (Figure 4-14). The correct TGC is achieved by moving sliders to the right to increase the gain for those regions close to the transducer

(Figure 4-15). Note the uniform image brightness compared with the image in Figure 4-14.

Although the TGC control affects sectional bands of the image according to depth, moving all of the TGC sliders by the same amount produces a change similar to an adjustment of the overall gain. Thus, gain and TGC controls are interdependent. If the gain is set too low or too high, the TGC sliders must then be positioned to the upper or lower range limits to compensate for the erroneous overall gain setting. In this circumstance, the ability to correctly fine-tune TGC is inhibited (Figure 4-16).

An additional consideration is the effect a change in transmit frequency has on the TGC control settings. Increased transmit frequency causes a higher rate of attenuation, requiring a greater slope of the gain curve. Decreased transmit frequency causes a

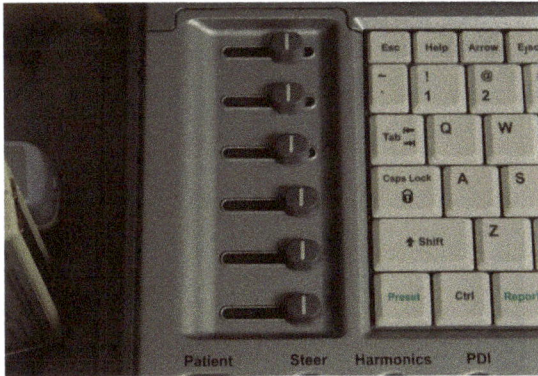

FIGURE 4-16. In this situation, overall gain should be increased and the sliders repositioned nearer to the midpoint of their ranges.

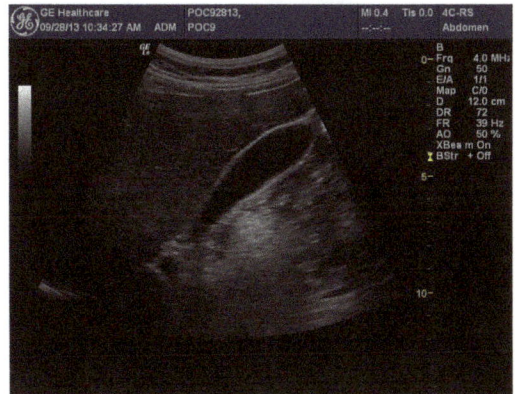

FIGURE 4-17. Single transmit focal zone set at a depth of 14 cm.

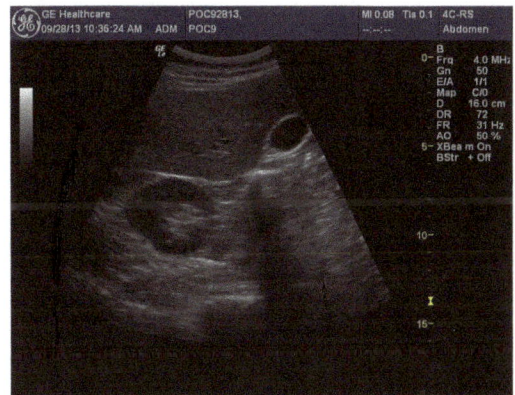

FIGURE 4-18. Single transmit focal zone set at a depth of 4 cm, denoted by hourglass-shaped indicator on right side of display.

lower rate of attenuation, requiring a less steep slope of the gain curve. Changes to overall gain and output power controls may also require adjustment of the TGC to maintain proper image brightness.

Reject

Reject control (also called threshold or suppression), by accepting only signals greater than a prescribed reference level (signal strength) for display, reduces low-amplitude noise in the image. Although the goal is to eliminate signals representing noise, weak signals from low-level reflectors along the beam path may also be eliminated if the reject control is set too high.

Transmit Focus

Lateral resolution is closely related to the beam width at any given point along the scan line. The B-mode control that minimizes the beam width at a specific depth is transmit focus. Focusing is achieved during beam formation by timed excitation of the elements that generate the pulsed sound wave. Only a single depth of focus can be prescribed for a transmitted beam. The region of increased intensity and narrowest beam width is called the focal zone. The center of the transmit focal zone is called the focal point, and is denoted on the real-time image by a small indicator located along the depth scale to the right of the display. Figure 4-17 shows the transmit focus set at a depth of approximately 4.5 cm. Changing the timed excitation of the transducer elements by adjusting

the transmit focus control alters the depth of focus to approximately 14 cm (Figure 4-18).

Lateral resolution is best at the focal point and then deteriorates with distance to either side of the focal point. Beyond the focal point the beam diverges rapidly, resulting in a wider sound beam and, therefore, reduced spatial detail due to degraded lateral resolution. Adjusting the depth of focus to reduce the beam width at one depth in the field of view therefore has the contradictory effect of degrading the lateral resolution at other depths (Figures 4-19 and 4-20).

Multiple transmit focus divides the scan line in segments in which each segment includes the focal point of a transmitted beam. Focal zones are distributed along the scan line as specified by the operator. Echoes from the separate transmitted beams,

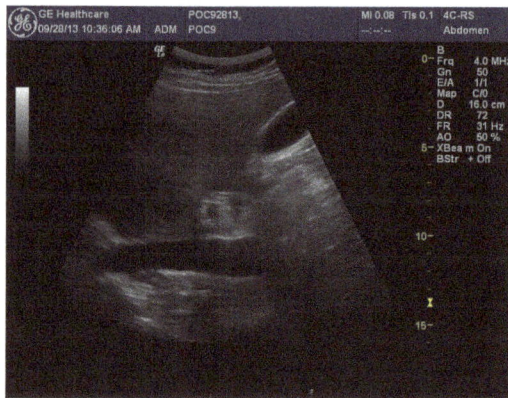

FIGURE 4-19. Single focal zone set at a depth of 14 cm. Loss of resolution occurs near the transducer.

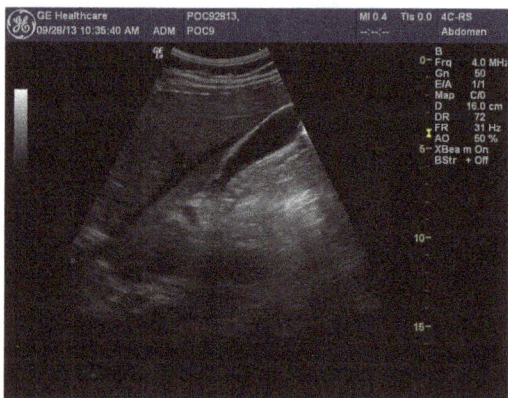

FIGURE 4-20. Single focal zone set at a depth of 4 cm. Loss of resolution occurs distal to the focal zone.

corresponding to the respective depth of focus, are overlaid to form a single scan line. If three transmit focal zones are selected, three separate transmit pulses are required to compose a single scan line. Therefore, each scan line takes generally three times as long to acquire the echo data, resulting in an approximate threefold reduction in the real-time frame rate. For example, a transducer operating at a maximum frame rate of 30 frames per second with a single focal zone would be reduced to 10 frames per second if three transmit focal zones were chosen (assuming the display depth is unchanged). The advantage of multiple transmit focal zones is that lateral resolution is improved throughout the designated portions of the scan line (Figure 4-21).

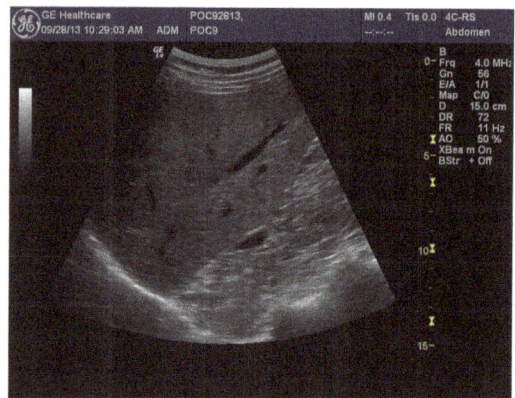

FIGURE 4-21. Four transmit focal zones distributed throughout the scan range indicated at right. Spatial resolution is improved at multiple depths along the scan line.

Optimize

Ultrasound transmission can be configured to enhance resolution or penetration, but not both. The parameters that can be adjusted include frequency, bandwidth, focal zones, and aperture. The optimize control allows the operator to select the desired emphasis, either resolution, penetration, or a balance between resolution and penetration. Adjustments are performed without input from the operator.

Sector Width

Phased array transducers produce images in the sector format. The width of the field of view is governed by the angle over which the transmit beam is swept. Adjustment of the sector angle is accomplished with the sector width control. A smaller (narrower) sector angle is advantageous for high scan line density and/or fast frame rate, with the consequence that the size of the field of view is reduced (visualization of nearby structures is sacrificed).

Zoom or Magnification

The display depth control is the fundamental means to alter image size and, when properly set, is an essential component of image optimization. Decreasing the display depth for the purpose of image magnification is appropriate in circumstances where either (1) the area of interest is fairly close to the transducer or (2) anatomy between the specific area of interest and the transducer must be included in the image.

If the display depth for deep-lying structures is decreased for the purpose of magnification, then the area of interest can be cut off at the bottom of the display. In this situation, the zoom control is the appropriate choice. The name of this control is vendor-specific, although most commonly referred to as "zoom," "res," or "mag." Some devices have two separate controls: one activates the "ROI cursor box" and one applies the magnification factor. Sometimes a single switch toggles between cursor on/cursor size/cursor position, which then selects the trackball to resize and to reposition the cursor box. Some systems offer the panning function, whereby the trackball scrolls the magnified image within the scanned field of view.

Dual Display

Activation of the dual display divides the monitor screen into two sections for the display of side-by-side 2D images. The split screen contains a frozen image and the "live" B-mode scan or two frozen images. The operator can toggle between the two screens to update with new images for comparison purposes. This is particularly useful in exam types that include a "pre" and "post" state, such as a venous duplex examination, in which a "non-compression" and a "compression" image of the same vessel are acquired.

Dynamic Range

Dynamic range expressed in dB represents the ratio of the largest to the smallest signal a system can process. Each returning echo is converted to an electrical signal that must be categorized according to its amplitude (strength) and stored as a digital value in the scan converter. The stored pixel value must then be translated to a shade of gray for display. Dynamic range alters the appearance of gray levels in the image, either emphasizing blacks and whites or extended intermediate grays.

Because the range of analog signal levels (approximately 100,000:1 or more) exceeds the number of discrete digital values available in the scan converter matrix (usually 0–255), signals must be partitioned according to a logarithmic scale. The dynamic range of the displayed image may equal the full dynamic range of the echo-induced signals or may be more restricted by excluding some high or low signals. In the latter case, the dynamic range is reduced. Low dynamic range improves image contrast, but usually with a loss of weaker echoes.

The operator control that varies the displayed dynamic range is called "dynamic range," "compression," or "log compression" (Figure 4-22). If the control is labeled "compression," an *increase* in value results

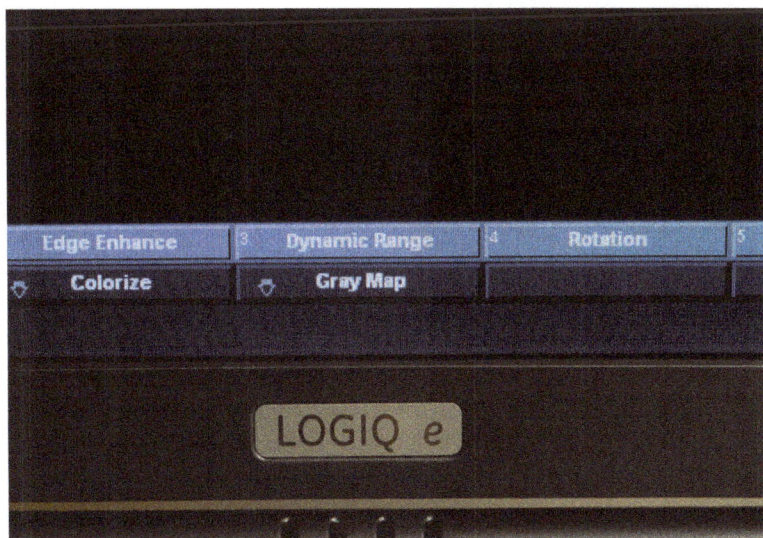

FIGURE 4-22. Dynamic range control.

is a *decrease* in dynamic range (dB is lowered). If the control is labeled "dynamic range," then an *increase* in value results in *increased* dynamic range (dB is raised). Sometimes this control is simplified by removing the dB label and allowing adjustment of dynamic range in incremental steps ranging from −3 to +3.

Displayed dynamic range may be described as wide or narrow. A wide dynamic range is considered to be 55–60 dB, while a narrow range is considered to be 40–45 dB (Figure 4-23). Wide dynamic range causes the image to appear low in contrast or "flat" because each gray level corresponds to large signal increments. Narrow dynamic range enhances the image contrast for a subset of the signal levels (often weak signals are excluded). Although there are theoretical differences

(A)

(B)

FIGURE 4-23. Effect on image contrast by changing dynamic range. (**A**) Sagittal image of the liver with "wide" dynamic range of 65 dB. (**B**) Sagittal image of the liver with "narrow" dynamic range of 45 dB.

regarding the contrast resolution of wide and narrow dynamic range images, in practice, personal preference is generally the determining factor. The ability to perceive informational content on the screen is also affected by the limited dynamic range of the monitor and the sensitivity of the human eye to distinguish slight differences in gray levels.

Frame Averaging

Persistence or frame averaging is a noise-reduction technique in which successive frames are temporarily stored in a buffer and then combined with the newly acquired frame for the real-time display. Commonly, two to four (or more) consecutive frames acquired over time are combined, with no change in overall displayed frame rate. Because noise is random at each pixel location and tends to cancel each other with time, while echoes from anatomical structures are consistent and repeatable, merging echo data from multiple scans of the field of view creates a less grainy appearance. However, fast moving objects become blurred in the image when persistence is increased.

Since frame averaging utilizes several frames acquired at different times, the technique is most effective for structures that are not in rapid motion, such as the liver or kidney. Fast moving structures, such as the heart, are poor candidates for frame averaging because of the large variation in spatial position over short-time intervals. Anatomical landmarks in successive frames are not superimposed at the same location in the averaged image and blurring occurs.

Temporal resolution is the ability to differentiate or resolve the dynamic motion of structures. Good temporal resolution is most important for structures with rapid movement. As frame averaging is increased, temporal resolution is degraded. For some applications such as imaging the liver, temporal resolution is not particularly important (because movement within the image is very slight) and the noise reduction achieved by frame averaging results in improved image quality. For other applications, such as the heart and blood vessels, the loss of temporal resolution is a significant consideration and far outweighs any advantage of frame averaging for noise reduction.

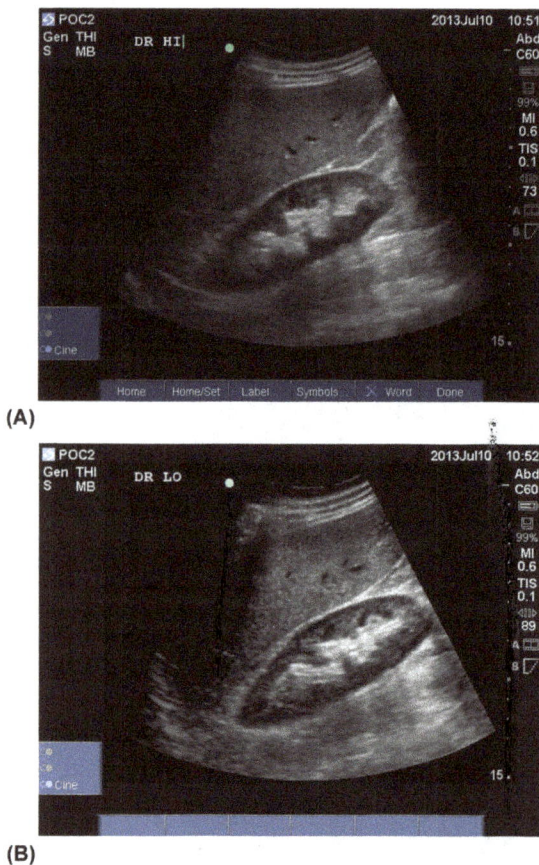

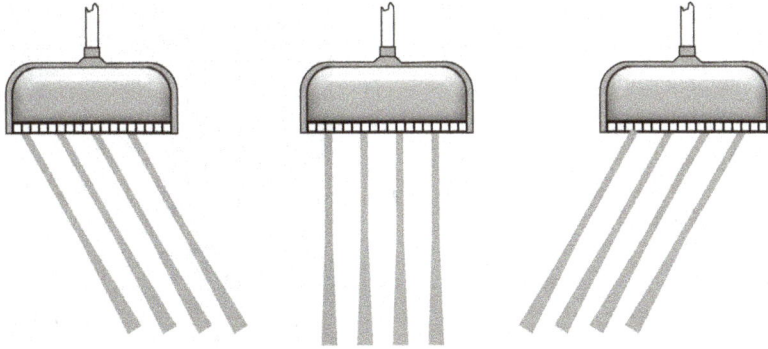

FIGURE 4-24. Spatial compounding. Three sequential frames obtained with different steered angles are combined to form a composite image.

Spatial Compounding

The amplitude of the echo-induced signal depends on the angle of incidence and the geometry of the boundary. Interrogating a specular reflector at normal incidence maximizes the intensity of the echo. During the examination the operator reorients the transducer, changing the relative beam direction with respect to an interface to maximize the reflectivity from that interface. In so doing, however, the less favorable beam orientation for other reflectors throughout the field of view causes their respective signals to be decreased. Spatial compounding, by acquiring multiple frames at different beam angles and combining the data, reduces acoustic noise while improving border definition of specular reflectors. Manufacturer's descriptors of this technique include sonoMB, sonoCT, cross beam, and multi-beam.

A group of elements in the array is stimulated to steer the beam at a specific angle. The active aperture is moved along the length of the array until all scan lines with that same beam angle are obtained, composing one frame of the field of view. The procedure is repeated for multiple beam angles, with each frame providing a unique angular sampling of the scanned tissue. Figure 4-24 shows a sequence of sampled frames using three distinct beam angles. The displayed image is a composite of the three most recently acquired steered frames. The signal for each pixel represents the collective weighted sum, the resultant from insonation at multiple beam directions. As each new frame is obtained, it is combined with the previous two frames held in memory. In this scheme, spatial averaging of the steered frames (each acquired with a unique scan angle) is accomplished in real time with little or no loss of frame rate.

Spatial compounding improves depiction of tissue boundaries and reduces noise variations (Figure 4-25).

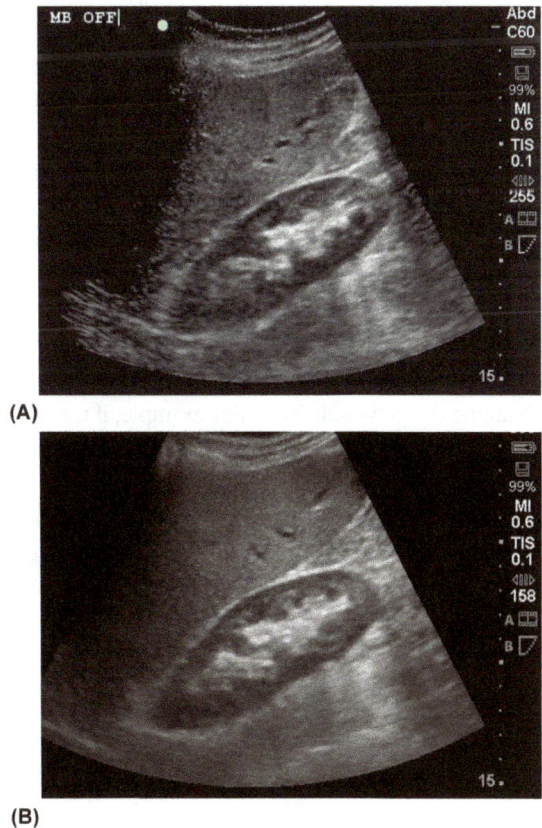

(A)

(B)

FIGURE 4-25. Effect of spatial compounding on image quality. (A) No spatial compounding. (B) Spatial compounding.

Attenuation artifacts, shadowing from strong reflectors and enhancement from weak reflectors, are less pronounced. Increasing the number of angles of insonification, and thus the number of combined frames, amplifies the compounding effect. However, since the image acquisition occurs over more frames separated in time, the potential for motion blur also increases.

Gray-Scale Mapping

The signal processing technique that alters displayed image contrast is gray-scale mapping. (Different from the dynamic range control, as gray-scale mapping occurs *after* echo data is stored in the scan converter matrix.) Each pixel is displayed uniformly as a particular shade of gray depending on the pixel value (Figure 4-26). Pixel values usually range from 0 to 255. That is, signal levels in the scan converter are distributed over 256 distinct numeric representations. The gray-scale map converts pixel values to brightness levels for image display. Since the number of brightness levels available on the monitor is less than the numeric range of pixel values, multiple signal levels must be associated with each gray level. Several gray-scale maps are available to change how this translation is performed (Figure 4-27). Selection of the gray-scale map does not alter the stored value in the scan converter; rather, it modifies how that pixel is displayed based on the stored value.

Pixels with similar values over a narrow range can be displayed with different degrees of brightness by changing the gray-scale map. For example, if the mid-range signals are judged to contain the most important

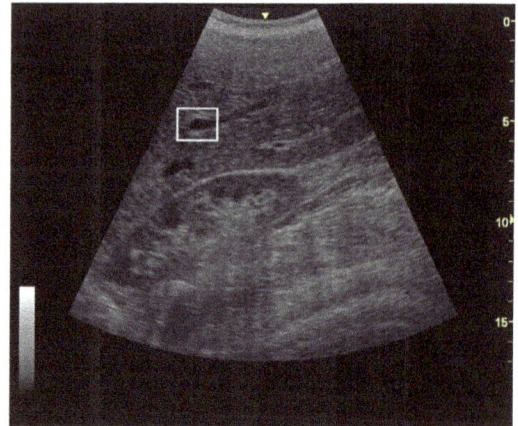

(A)

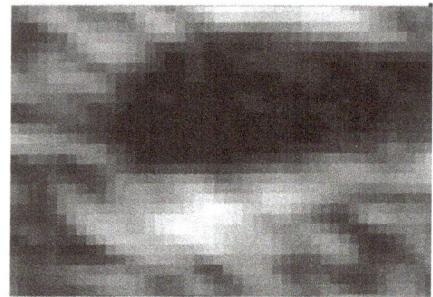

(B)

FIGURE 4-26. Pixels as components of a digital image. (**A**) Sonogram of the liver. (**B**) Magnification of the B-mode image (which includes a blood vessel) to illustrate individual pixels with varying levels of brightness.

echo data, the available shades of gray may be concentrated so that more shades are assigned to the mid-range signal levels than for the high or low signals. Contrast is improved within the limited mid-range because the shades of gray are distributed over contracted signal

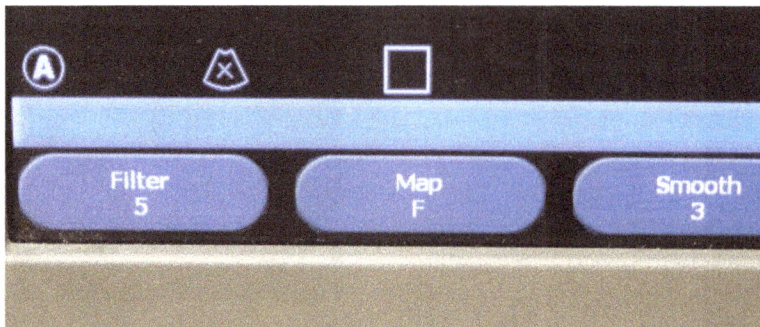

FIGURE 4-27. Gray-scale map control.

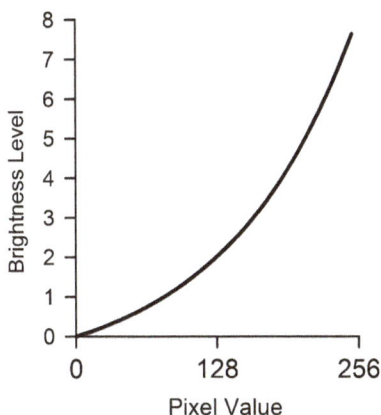

FIGURE 4-28. Gray-scale map in which contrast enhancement is applied for high signal levels.

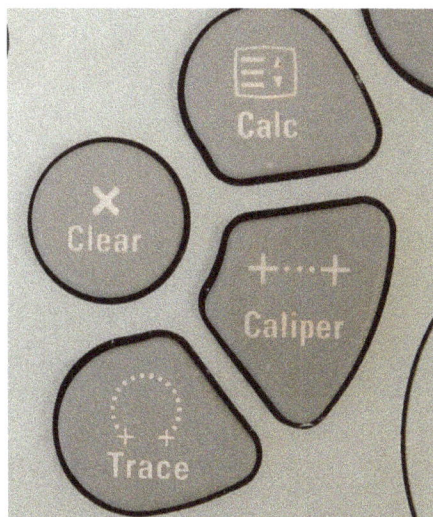

FIGURE 4-29. Measurements are performed using the caliper function.

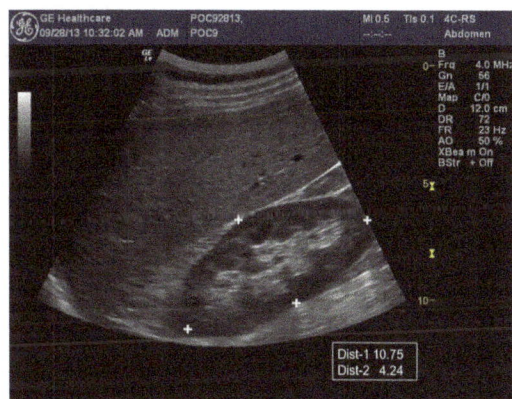

FIGURE 4-30. Sagittal image of the kidney with two sets of calipers which measure the sagittal and A-P (anterior-posterior) dimensions.

levels (the range of pixel values associated with a particular shade of gray is reduced). Each gray-scale map is designed to emphasize a specific segment of echo signal levels (Figure 4-28). Individual maps are typically labeled A through Z, and often AA, BB, etc.

Measurements

Measurements of linear distance, circumference, and area are routinely performed using sonography. Most ultrasound systems have two options for making measurements. The first utilizes a software calculation package, which is application-specific (obstetric, cardiac, vascular, etc.). The application preset determines, along with control default settings, the appropriate calculation package. The measurement package guides the operator through the data acquisition process and, ultimately, creates a report of the results. The second option is a stand-alone measurement of linear distance, area, or circumference. Measurements are made by pressing the caliper button and positioning the on-screen cursor with the trackball (Figure 4-29). A "select" key activates each caliper cursor alternately, so that the position of each is adjusted independently. Often, multiple sets of calipers can be displayed on the screen simultaneously (Figure 4-30).

A manual, single measurement, not part of the calculation package, is frequently performed for structures such as the gallbladder wall or common bile duct. Manual measurements are also necessary

in circumstances where no preprogrammed calculation software is available (e.g., the dimensions of the pancreas or thickness of the abdominal wall). Often, single on-the-fly measurements are obtained in cardiac imaging for a quick estimation of left atrial size or left ventricle wall thickness.

For accurate linear measurements, the caliper position must be carefully chosen. Focus and display depth should be optimized for the organ of interest. The gain or TGC are reduced to minimize

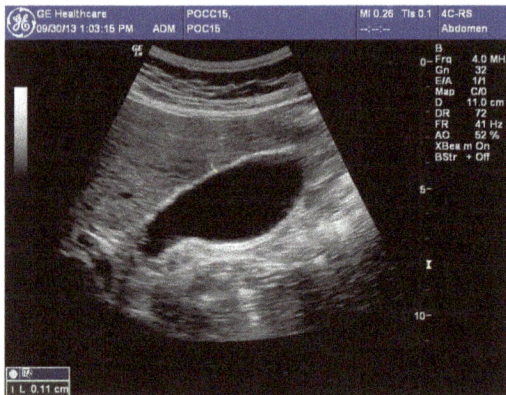

FIGURE 4-31. Measurement of the thickness of the gallbladder wall. The displayed image has been magnified to facilitate the placement of cursors.

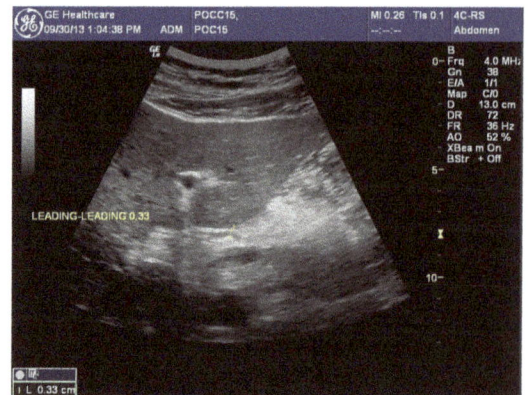

FIGURE 4-32. Common bile duct measured as 0.33 cm using the leading edge-to-leading edge technique.

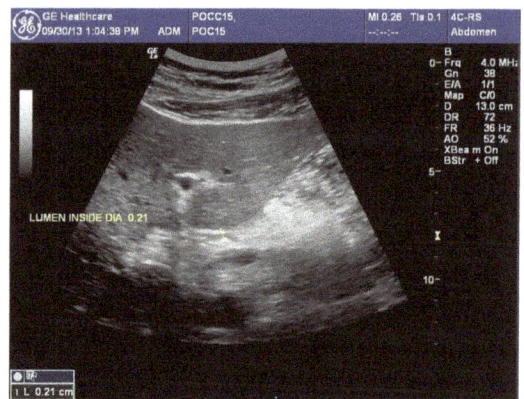

FIGURE 4-33. Common bile duct measured as 0.21 cm using the trailing edge-to-leading edge technique.

any ring-down artifact that might create an artifactually "thicker" interface such as the gallbladder wall (Figure 4-31). Traditionally, most linear measurements were made "leading edge to leading edge." The belief was that the leading edge of a reflecting interface was more faithfully reproduced than the trailing edge and is relatively independent of equipment settings for output power, gain, or TGC. Therefore, measurements of the fetal biparietal diameter were made from the outer edge of the skull bone to the inner edge of the bone on the opposite side of the head. Measurements for the common bile duct were performed in the same way.

Today, with the continual improvement in image quality, the calipers are generally placed on the outer or inner boundary of the organ without regard to the leading edge technique. Measurement of fetal biparietal diameter still requires the leading edge-to-leading edge method. However this is not necessarily attributed to better accuracy, but rather because the fetal growth charts were developed based on this technique. If the outer-to-outer technique were now used, the growth charts would need to be revised.

Nevertheless, sonographic measurements must conform to the guidelines of the institution (e.g., leading edge to leading edge or other methodology). The difference in measurement technique can result in small, although sometimes significant, error (Figures 4-32 and 4-33).

Circumference and area measurements, whether performed within a calculation package or as stand-alone, can be executed with free-hand tracing or with the ellipse tool. The free-hand tracing method positions one caliper at a start point and then the operator manually draws, freehand, the boundary around the organ or structure. This can be somewhat awkward and success depends to a large extent on the artistic ability and motor control of the operator. (Figure 4-34) The second method, which is available on many systems, employs an ellipse tool. The ellipse is positioned on screen by locating two reference points (with calipers) until the ellipse coincides with the borders of the structure to be measured. If the structure is near circular in shape, the measurement

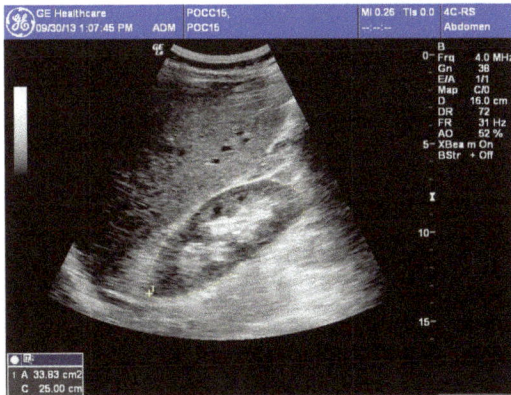

FIGURE 4-34. Area and circumference of the right kidney measured with the free-hand trace tool.

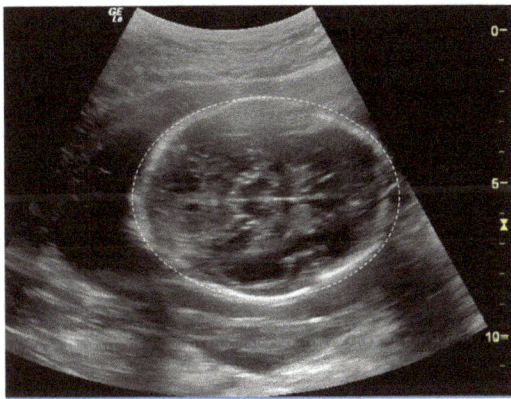

FIGURE 4-35. Circumference of the fetal head measured with the ellipse tool.

is complete at this point. If the structure is ovoid in shape, a third control allows the shape of the ellipse to be stretched into an oval. The oval ellipse is then manipulated by the trackball until it is superimposed on the structure (Figure 4-35).

APPLICATION PRESETS

Manufacturers have developed initial, practical operator control settings for each type of examination, called application presets. The same operator controls are manipulated during sonographic examination of the liver, kidneys, heart, carotid arteries, uterus and ovaries, leg veins, neonatal brain, fetus, breast, and thyroid gland. However, the settings of these controls vary significantly depending on the exam type. The organ may be fluid-filled like the gallbladder or homogeneous tissue like the spleen. The structures may be stationary or rapidly moving. Often, the sound beam must first pass through the chest wall or abdominal wall or a full urinary bladder. At times the operator must scan between ribs or through the bone of the skull or image 1 cm beneath the skin surface. For each of these situations, there is a common set of hardware choices and control settings that are well defined. This group of settings becomes the default configuration for the exam-specific application preset.

As an example, consider an ultrasound examination of an adult heart. Requirements for imaging this organ include the need to scan between ribs (sector transducer), a relatively low transmit frequency to penetrate the chest wall, tissue harmonic imaging, and high frame rate. Settings for sector width, power, persistence, number of focal zones, and gray-scale map are required. The heart, composed of muscular walls and fluid-filled chambers, requires a unique TGC curve, since it is not homogeneous like the liver.

As another example, consider a transabdominal GYN exam. The transducer must provide a medium-sized field of view (curvilinear array) and the sound beam must penetrate the abdominal wall, including fat layers (influences the choice of transmit frequency). The beam path includes the full urinary bladder, where there is very little attenuation. The organs of interest lie deep within the pelvis, so excellent detail at a deep scan depth (focal depth) is required. A high frame rate is not required, which enables frame averaging, spatial compounding, and multiple transmit focal zones to be applied for improved image quality. A wide field of view is needed near the transducer to evaluate the anterior bladder wall (a sector would not be the ideal choice). For this examination, the transducer, TGC, transmit frequency, persistence, and number of focal zones are very different from that of the heart exam described above.

Default values for each application preset are installed at time of manufacture. Typically, an ultrasound machine is preprogrammed with a generic listing of common examinations with corresponding subsets. Default values for each preset represent typical values for each control, tailored to each type of exam. Most ultrasound systems allow user-programmable application presets. For example, if the operator prefers to begin an abdominal exam with a different display depth, he/she can create a new preset (with a different name) employing the new depth setting. The same practice applies for other parameters such as dynamic range, gray-scale map, and color map. Multiple operators can each configure their own presets, if desired.

Within each exam type, optimal control settings vary from patient to patient based on age, size, weight, body habitus, and disease process. Therefore, the application preset is only a starting point. The operator must either confirm the correct settings or make adjustments in the controls as necessary to produce an optimum image. Often, these controls must be adjusted frequently as the transducer is moved into different scan planes during the course of the actual examination.

Typically, the exam preset selection control generates a hierarchical drop-down menu listing the top level of exam presets. The general examination type is then selected from a list of available exam presets.

OPERATIONAL MODES

Advances in instrumentation have created additional operational modes beyond traditional B-mode imaging. These new imaging techniques include extended field of view, tissue harmonic imaging, elastography, 3D, and 4D imaging. A unique method called M-mode, which characterizes the movement of reflectors, is also included in this section.

Extended Field of View

The advantages of real-time ultrasound include excellent temporal resolution (high frame rate), focusing using multiple-element arrays, and freedom to position the transducer. Real-time field of view is limited in size by transducer width (linear array), sector scanning angle (phased array), or radius of curvature (curvilinear array). To establish spatial relationships throughout a large region, the operator must compose a mental picture of the anatomy by acquiring several, small field of view frames throughout the area of interest.

Extended field of view real-time ultrasound combines successive frames to form a panoramic image as the transducer is moved across the patient. Extended field of view real-time imaging employs computer analysis of image features to determine transducer location without sensors or an articulating arm. The field of view of the panoramic image is larger than the field of view of a single real-time frame. Sonograms of a forearm and a neck acquired with extended field of view are shown in Figures 4-36 and 4-37.

The fidelity of registration process is corrupted by actions that reduce image feature similarity. The primary factors that can cause artifacts are large-scale

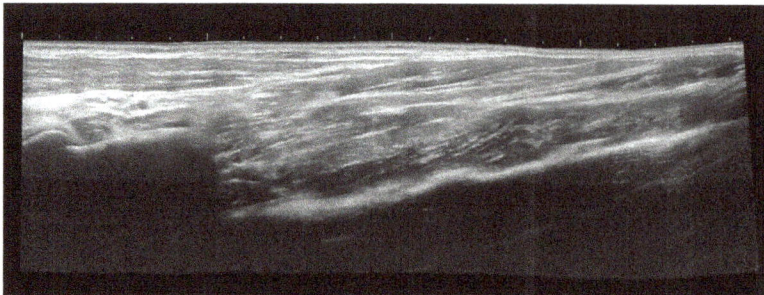

FIGURE 4-36. Extended field of view of a forearm.

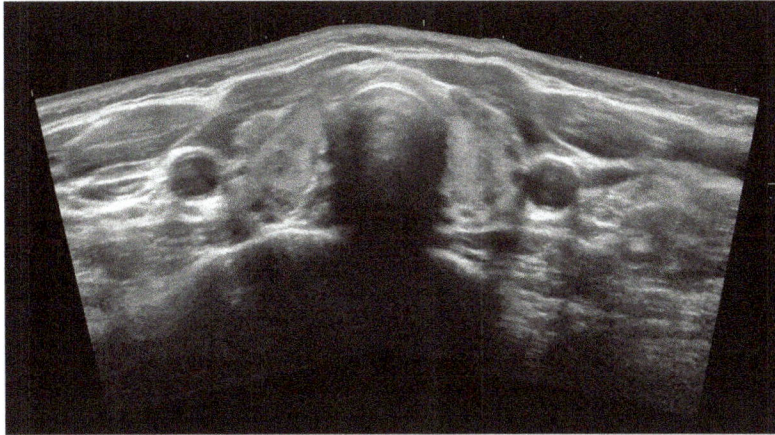

FIGURE 4-37. Extended field of view of a neck in the transverse plane.

tissue motion and off-plane rotation. Tissue motion contributes to the displacement of common image features and results in improper registration of the current frame. Off-plane rotation shifts the imaging plane at an angle into or out of the plane of the reference image. The sampled anatomical region is changed, which eliminates common image features. Small-scale off-plane rotation inherent in free-hand scanning is usually tolerated in extended field of view imaging.

Tissue Harmonic Imaging

Tissue harmonic imaging (THI) is an imaging technique that relies on the detection of the second harmonic frequency by the exclusion of the transmitted fundamental frequency. Even though the second harmonic signal is weaker than traditional echo ranging utilizing the fundamental frequency, contrast is often improved by the suppression of interfering signals from clutter and multiangle scattering.

The pulsed sound wave is transmitted with intensity sufficient to cause nonlinear propagation through tissue. At the point of transmission, only the fundamental frequency (and the associated bandwidth) is present, but as the sound moves away from the transducer into the body, the pulsed wave becomes distorted with the introduction of the second harmonic frequency. The second harmonic frequency continues

to form until intensity is reduced and linear propagation is established. This creates a region within the ultrasonic field where second harmonic frequencies are present. An echo from a reflector within this region is composed of both the fundamental transmitted frequency and the second harmonic frequency. At reception, the second harmonic frequency is isolated from the fundamental frequency and then processed for display. As an example, the transmitted frequency is set at 2 MHz, and then the image is formed using the second harmonic frequency of 4 MHz. Since clutter and multiangle scattering occurs predominantly at the fundamental frequency, these noise sources are eliminated in the tissue harmonic image.

The transmit frequency control on some scanners also activates tissue harmonic imaging. As the control continues to be increased beyond the highest transmit frequency for the fundamental imaging mode, the system automatically switches into harmonic imaging. In harmonic mode, the transmit frequency may be indicated as "H1, H2," or by some other labeling scheme (Figure 4-38).

Elastography

Elastography detects the relative tissue displacement between precompression (no palpation) and compression (palpation) measured by ultrasound. The amount of force required to cause a given

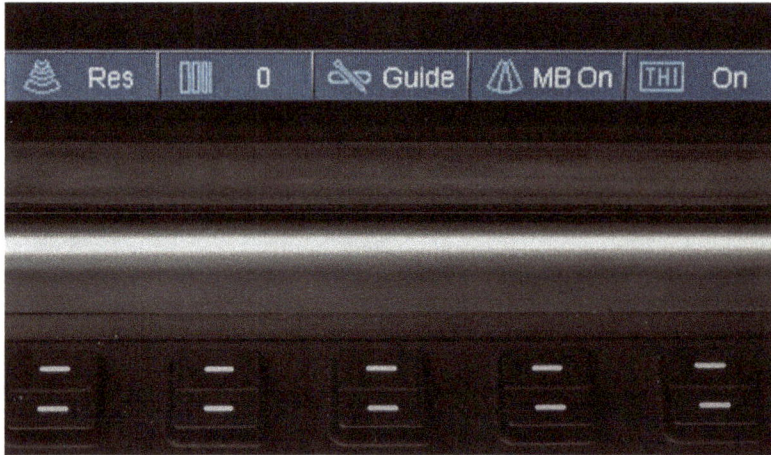

FIGURE 4-38. Tissue harmonic imaging control on a point-of-care ultrasound system.

displacement depends on the tissue type. Removal of the force restores the elastic tissue to the original shape and dimensions. The parameter that describes how likely the tissue maintains its shape when the force is applied is called stiffness. Fat, glandular tissue, carcinoma, and fibrous tissue have different degrees of stiffness.

Ultrasound determines the locations of reflectors under conditions of palpation and no palpation. The difference in position yields the displacement caused by the force. A 2D quantitative map of tissue stiffness is compiled. Dual display of elasticity and B-mode images is shown side by side in a split screen format. The measured stiffness and the relative lesion size in B-mode versus elasticity images may allow tissue differentiation. Elastography of the breast may more accurately identify lesions for biopsy.

Three-Dimensional Imaging

In 2D imaging, the operator must mentally form a three-dimensional (3D) impression of the anatomy from a series of acquired B-mode images. This process is time consuming, subjective, and inconsistent. Depending on operator proficiency, spatial relationships are often distorted or misrepresented. In 3D imaging, the spatial relationships of structures within a scanned volume are represented by an image or a set of images. Following data collection, echo information is processed for display as a static image. Real-time scanning of the tissue volume is called four-dimensional (4D) imaging and is discussed in the following section.

In free-hand scanning, the transducer is moved manually across the patient without any position sensing device. The transducer movement must be uniform and conform to the predefined scanning geometry. Deviations from the assumed scanning motion introduce geometric distortion in the reconstructed volume. This technique is limited to qualitative assessment, since measurements of distance, area, and volume are generally not accurate.

A 3D transducer mechanically moves a multiple-element crystal array across the beam port to interrogate a volume. The direction of movement is perpendicular to the crystal row. The crystal array allows electronic steering of the beam within the plane defined by the mechanical position of the crystal array. At each position along the arc, multiple scan lines form a 2D image. A series of 2D images are acquired during movement of the array, which establishes the sampled 3D volume. The crystal array is encased in fluid within the transducer housing to provide good energy transmission into tissue.

The most common method to form the 3D volume data set is voxel-based reconstruction. A voxel is a 3D picture element with length, width, and thickness.

The dimensions in each direction are not necessarily the same. Each pixel in the set of 2D images is placed at the proper location within the volume. If a voxel was not sampled by a 2D image, then the value for that voxel is calculated by interpolation using the values from neighboring voxels.

After reconstruction the 3D volume is viewed interactively using computer graphics. Information is extracted from the volume data set and then displayed. The process of selecting and manipulating data for visualization is called rendering. Three types of rendering form 3D images for display: multiplanar formatting, surface rendering, and volume rendering.

The 3D data set is composed of voxels that are stacked together as a pile of bricks. Similar to isolating the bricks that comprise one layer, the operator can view a single plane in the 3D volume. Imagine that the pile of bricks can be cut in any orientation and a single layer of bricks extracted. Following their removal, another single layer of bricks with the same orientation but one layer offset from the first is extracted. The 3D volume can be rotated so that the operator can view its contents along any line of sight. Once the line of sight is established, the visualized 2D images are formed using one layer of voxels in the plane perpendicular to this line of sight. In this manner, successive parallel plane images are generated at equal intervals along the operator's line of sight, and the operator can scroll through the set of 2D images. Typically, three orthogonal planes are displayed simultaneously with indicators regarding their orientation and intersection (Figure 4-39).

Surface rendering depicts the surface of organs or other structures for display. The boundaries of the structure are identified by the operator or by computer contouring. The points within the boundary are interconnected by a wire mesh formed in triangular or polygonal segments. Once the surface is established, the texture and lighting are changed depending on the operator's viewing perspective (Figure 4-40).

Volume rendering allows a 3D view of the scanned tissue. The viewing direction must first be established. Then, a set of parallel rays is directed through the 3D volume. Each ray corresponds to one pixel in the volume-rendered image. The voxels encountered along each ray are identified, the values are

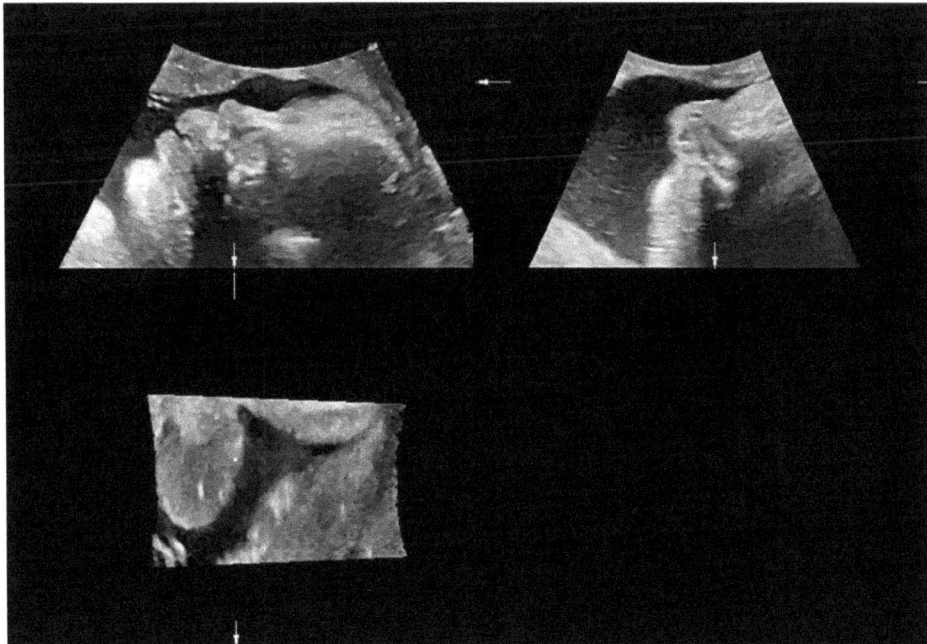

FIGURE 4-39. Three orthogonal planes in 3D imaging of the fetus.

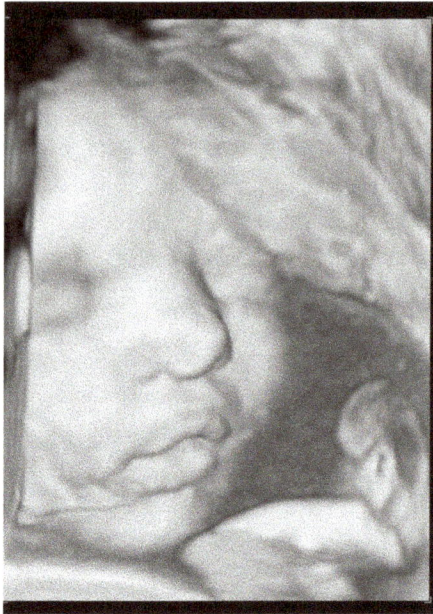

FIGURE 4-40. Surface rendering of the fetus.

multiplied by factors, and their products are summed to obtain the final value for that ray (pixel). The array of pixels is configured in a 2D projection image. One common approach is to generate a maximum intensity projection image. This type of volume rendering retains only the maximum voxel value along each ray. All other voxel values are excluded.

The translucent/opacity rendering technique weights the voxel values along each ray by opacity and color factors. The opacities, shades, and colors encountered along the ray are blended to produce the final pixel color and luminance in the 2D projection image. The opacity and color factors are adjustable to depict the desired anatomical structures. Volume rendering has been very successful in the display of fetal and vascular anatomy.

4D Ultrasound

Display of a surface-rendered plane or multiple planes of the sampled volume in real time is called 4D ultrasound. The fourth dimension of time is combined with volumetric sampling to depict the dynamic spatial relationships of structures in three dimensions. Mechanically steered multiple-element

arrays have been developed to rapidly acquire volumetric data. Since fewer scan lines are acquired compared with 3D ultrasound, some loss in spatial resolution occurs in 4D ultrasound. Also, resolution deteriorates with distance from the transducer (lower scan line density). Different transducer types including curvilinear, linear, and endocavity are available.

M-Mode

The spatial locations of reflectors along a single line of sight are combined with the time of observation to form a two dimensional recording called an M-mode trace. Using a high pulse repetition frequency, the transmitted beam is repeatedly directed along a single sampling direction. The detected echoes from each transmitted pulse are registered with respect to axial distance from the transducer (echo wavetrain), and multiple transmitted pulses provide the temporal changes in each reflector's position. A time sweep of the sequential echo wavetrains proceeds across the screen at a constant rate. Tick marks show the timing interval. The sweep speed can be varied to improve temporal resolution or to extend the plot over a longer time interval. Control of sweep rate may be by setting a numerical value or by selection of slow, medium, or fast. Straight lines on the display correspond to stationary reflectors, whereas fluctuating waveforms indicate moving reflectors (Figure 4-41). *The information content of the M-mode trace includes:*

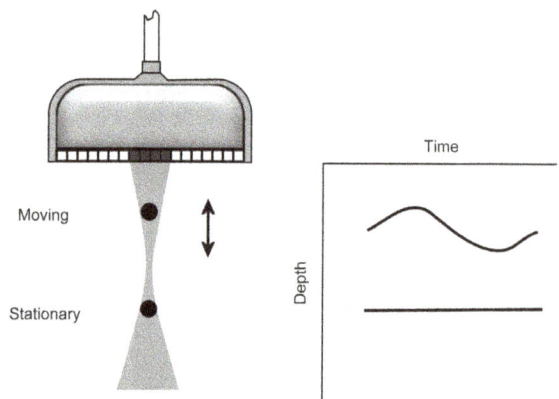

FIGURE 4-41. The axial position of each reflector along the beam path is repeatedly sampled to detect motion.

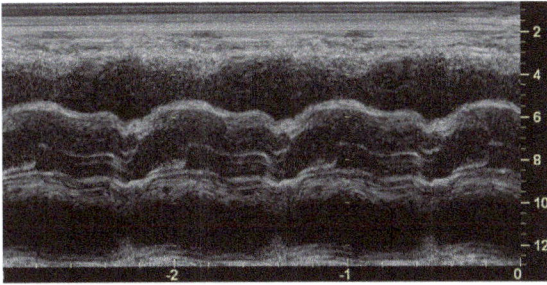

FIGURE 4-42. M-mode trace of the aortic valve.

reflector depth, reflectivity (gray-scale shading), relative positions of the reflectors along the sampling direction, and change in axial position of each reflector with time. Motion in the lateral direction is not known because sampling is limited to one line of sight. High pulse repetition frequency allows very rapid motion to be characterized faithfully.

The M-mode trace in Figure 4-42 illustrates strong specular reflection from the walls of the aortic root and left atrium, and the low amplitude tissue scatterers. The sweep rate can change the pattern of the M-mode trace, dependent on the speed of the moving interface.

When combined with B-mode imaging, the M-mode sampling direction can be specified with respect to the visualized anatomy. This facilitates assessment of the moving structures of interest and provides correlation between the two scanning modes. The screen is divided into two sections to

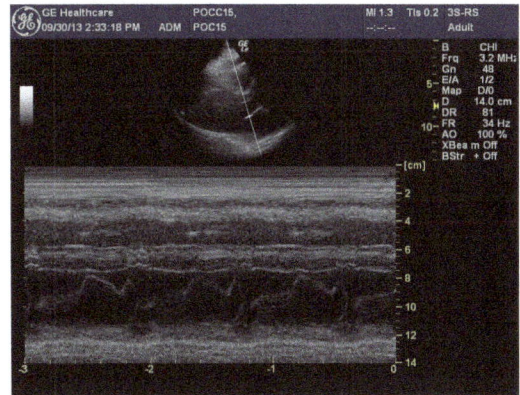

FIGURE 4-43. Combined M-mode and B-mode imaging. The B-mode image facilitates the designation of the sampling direction for M-mode.

show the B-mode image and the M-mode trace. A line cursor is placed on the gray-scale image to designate the sampling direction for the M-mode acquisition (Figure 4-43). The B-mode frame rate is reduced while the M-mode trace is collected.

References

Hedrick WR: Technology for diagnostic sonography, St. Louis, 2013, Elsevier.

Hedrick WR, Hykes DL, Starchman DE: Ultrasound physics and instrumentation, ed 4, St. Louis, 2005, Elsevier.

Kremkau FW: Diagnostic ultrasound: principles and instruments, ed 8, Philadelphia, 2011, WB Saunders.

Zagzebski JA: Essentials of ultrasound physics, St Louis, 1996, Mosby-Year Book.

5

Doppler Principles and Displays

KEY TERMS

Aliasing
Beat frequency
Color flow imaging
Color map
Color velocity scale
Color wall filter
Combined Doppler mode
Cutoff frequency
Doppler angle

Doppler effect
Doppler shift frequency
Doppler spectral waveform
Maximum velocity waveform
Packet size (ensemble length)
Power Doppler imaging
Spectral analysis
Velocity scale

INTRODUCTION

The ability to identify flow patterns and measure flow velocities is one of the most important functions of diagnostic ultrasound. The sonographer must understand the factors that contribute to the Doppler information displayed on the monitor. Most of what we discuss in this chapter applies to both spectral Doppler and color flow imaging, since each mode is governed by the Doppler equation and is ultimately subject to the same factors.

THE DOPPLER EFFECT

The Doppler effect is the observed change in frequency of a transmitted wave due to the relative motion between the source of the sound and the receiver or observer. Doppler ultrasound is a valuable tool because this methodology detects the presence, direction, velocity, and time variation of blood flow within blood vessels and in the heart. Several types of Doppler devices are available. Although each relies on the Doppler effect to detect motion, the manner in which flow information is acquired, processed, and displayed distinguishes one type of instrument from another. Some scanners offer several Doppler modes, which are selectable by the user. The most basic (inexpensive) systems offer only a single option for the Doppler mode (velocity analysis or two-dimension Doppler imaging, i.e. color flow).

The apparent frequency change produced by the Doppler effect is based on the relative motion between the source of sound and the observer, regardless of which is moving and which is stationary. When a police car with siren blaring passes a pedestrian, the audible sound is heard as a change in frequency or *pitch* as the vehicle approaches (the frequency appears to be higher) while the frequency of the retreating vehicle after it passes is observed to be lower. In the above illustration, the sound source is the moving vehicle, while the receiver or observer is the stationary pedestrian.

Imagine a situation in which an observer is standing in a boat in the middle of a lake. If the wind is blowing at a constant rate from the north and the waves all have the same distance between peaks (same wavelength), the stationary boat will encounter the same number of wave crests each second (constant frequency) as are produced by the wind. If the boat begins traveling in a northerly direction, *into* the wind, the wave crests are encountered more frequently. The observer standing in the boat sees an increase in the wave frequency, although, in actuality, the frequency of the cresting waves has not changed. If the boat turns around and begins heading south, this time *with* the wind (away from the source of the waves), fewer crests are seen, and to the observer the frequency appears to decrease. As the boat moves faster in either direction, the difference between the actual and observed frequencies becomes greater. The only circumstance in which these "transmitted" and "observed" frequencies are the same is when the boat is stationary.

A stationary observer views the same number of pressure waves as are emitted by the stationary source (Figure 5-1). However, the relative motion between the sound source and the receiver distorts the pattern of symmetric wavefronts and the observed frequency increases or decreases, depending upon the direction of movement. The change or difference in frequency between the transmitted frequency and the received frequency, caused by the motion, is the Doppler shift frequency (often abbreviated as "Doppler shift" or "Doppler frequency"). In the example of the police siren above, the frequency appears higher to the stationary observer as the car approaches. In this case, the relative motion of the source and the receiver is toward one another. As the police car passes and travels away from the observer, the frequency appears to decrease, since the relative movement between the source and the observer is away from one another.

When considering a sound wave produced by a piezoelectric transducer, the sound source remains stationary while the moving "receiver" could be blood cells or another moving structure, such as a heart valve. The echo from the moving reflector is then observed with a Doppler shift frequency by the stationary transducer, which is now the receiver.

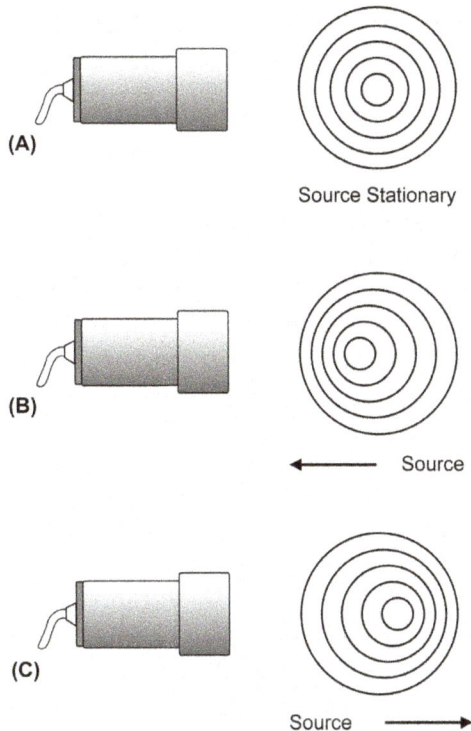

FIGURE 5-1. The Doppler effect. (**A**) Stationary sound source and receiver, the observed frequency is the same as the frequency emitted by the sound source. (**B**) Sound source moving toward the receiver, the observed frequency is higher than the actual frequency emitted by the sound source. (**C**) Sound source moving away from the receiver, the observed frequency is lower than the actual frequency emitted by the sound source.

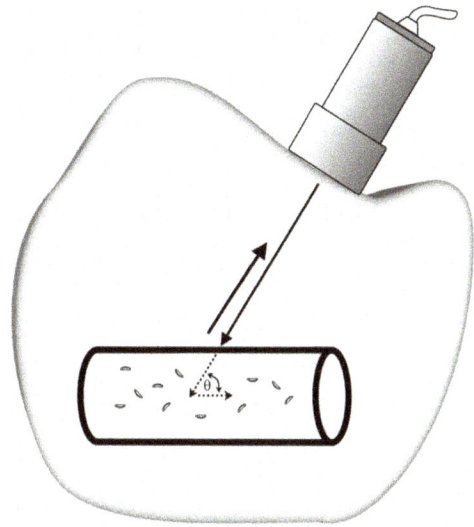

FIGURE 5-2. Doppler ultrasound detection of reflector velocity. The Doppler angle θ is defined by the reflector path with respect to the transmitted beam.

Doppler Shift Equation

The magnitude of the Doppler shift frequency depends on how rapidly the sound source, the receiver, or both are moving in relation to one another. An increase in the relative velocity between the source and the receiver causes a greater deviation from the transmitted frequency. *Indeed, this is the rationale behind why we perform the Doppler examination.* The Doppler shift frequency (f_D) produced by a moving reflector is calculated from the equation:

$$f_D = \frac{2vf}{c}\cos\theta \qquad 5\text{-}1$$

where c is the acoustic velocity of tissue, f is the transmitted frequency, v is the velocity of the interface,

and θ is the angle between the path of reflector movement and the direction of beam propagation (called the Doppler angle or angle to flow) as illustrated in Figure 5-2. Note that the letter "c" in the Doppler equation represents the velocity of sound in tissue instead of the usual "v" for velocity. In this mathematical symbolism, the character "v" is reserved for the velocity of the flowing blood. The number 2 in the equation represents two separate (and equal) Doppler shifts that occur in Doppler ultrasound. The first Doppler shift occurs between the stationary sound source, the transducer, and the "observer," the moving blood cells. The second Doppler shift takes place as the moving blood cells (now the sound source) reflect the sound wave back to the stationary transducer, which now becomes the receiver.

As a reflector moves directly toward a 5-MHz transducer at a velocity of 50 cm/s, the angle to flow is 0 degrees and the observed frequency is 5,003,247 Hz, corresponding to a Doppler shift frequency of 3247 Hz above the original transmitted frequency (Figure 5-3). If the flow is away from that transducer at 50 cm/s, the observed frequency is 4,996,753 Hz or 3247 Hz below the original transmitted frequency. The Doppler angle

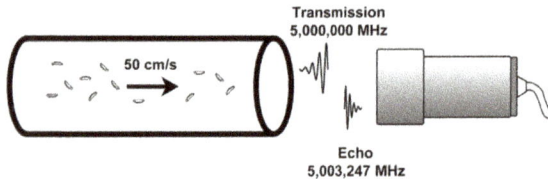

FIGURE 5-3. Received echo frequency is 3247 Hz above the transmitted frequency when the flow velocity is 50 cm/s toward the transducer. The transmitted frequency is 5 MHz and the Doppler angle θ is 0 degrees.

gives the component of the velocity along the direction of propagation for the ultrasound beam. If the Doppler angle is increased from 0 to 30 degrees, the Doppler shift frequency is 2.8 kHz instead of the 3.2 kHz obtained for parallel incidence. For a given reflector velocity, the Doppler shift frequency decreases as the Doppler angle is increased (Figure 5-4).

No Doppler shift frequency occurs at a 90-degree angle of incidence (cosine theta in the Doppler equation is equal to zero for an incident angle of 90 degrees). In practice, the signal never disappears completely. Because the beam has a finite width, some

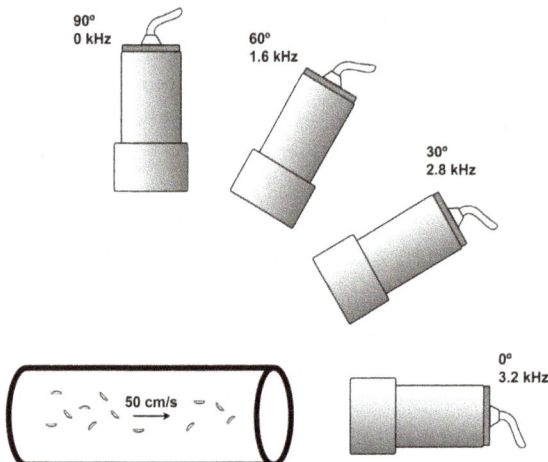

FIGURE 5-4. Doppler shift frequency from reflectors moving at a velocity of 50 cm/s versus Doppler angle. The transmit frequency is 5 MHz. The Doppler shift frequency is 3.2 kHz at 0 degrees, 2.8 Hz at 30 degrees, and 1.6 kHz at 60 degrees. No Doppler shift frequency is observed at 90 degrees.

portion of the beam impinges at an angle that is not perpendicular to the motion. Beam divergence tends to amplify this effect, especially in the region beyond the beam's focal point.

Velocity Determination

The acoustic velocity is assumed to remain constant at a value of 1540 m/s for soft tissue. The observed change in frequency occurs because the sound beam encounters a moving structure between the source and the detector. The Doppler equation predicts that an increase in reflector velocity results in a greater Doppler shift frequency. *If the Doppler shift frequency and angle to flow are known, the velocity of the moving reflectors can be calculated.* In practice, the transmitted and received frequencies are first measured, and then processed to find the resultant Doppler shift frequency. The instrument accomplishes these steps autonomously without operator intervention. *However, the Doppler angle to flow must be determined by the sonographer with manual input to the scanner for the correct display of flow velocity.*

Uncertainty in the measurement of the Doppler angle, particularly at large angles, introduces error in the velocity computation. The exact angle to flow is much more of a consideration when evaluating blood vessels than in the heart due to differences in acoustic access. In vascular applications, the process of *angle correction* (angle measurement) must be performed by the sonographer in order to achieve an accurate estimation of flow velocity. At a Doppler angle to flow of 60 degrees, the resultant Doppler shift is only half that with a Doppler angle of 0 degrees. The angle to flow must be measured as accurately as possible, because a 5-degree deviation for a 60-degree angle to flow (frequently used when examining blood vessels) introduces an 18% error in the measurement of flow velocity.

Conversely, when the beam is near parallel to flow (as is frequently the case in the heart), the Doppler angle to flow is assumed to be 0 degrees and no angle correction is performed. At a Doppler angle to flow near 0 degrees, a 5-degree inaccuracy in the angle results in only a 1% error in the calculation of flow velocity. A 10-degree error in the estimation of Doppler angle to flow results in a velocity error of less than 10%. In practice, the angle of insonation is assumed to be 0 degrees in cardiac applications and no "angle correction" is performed.

Doppler signals from superficial blood vessels (e.g., the carotids) should generally not be acquired at angles greater than 60 degrees, due to the increased potential of error as the Doppler angle approaches 90 degrees. Regardless of the angle, care should be taken in vascular applications to measure the angle to flow as accurately as possible.

Scattering from Blood

For Doppler measurements of blood flow, red blood cells (RBCs) act as Rayleigh scatterers. The RBC has a diameter of 7 μ (much smaller than the wavelength of the sound wave, usually 0.2–0.5 mm) and thus meets the condition for Rayleigh scattering. Rayleigh scattering exhibits very strong frequency dependence (proportional to the fourth power of the frequency). Therefore, the intensity of the scattered ultrasound energy increases dramatically as the transmitted frequency increases.

The intensity of the scattered sound also depends on the number of RBCs and thus the quantity of blood in the sample volume. Because the scattering from blood is small compared with echoes produced by soft tissue interfaces, blood-filled vessels appear to be echo-free on the B-mode image. To enhance scattering and, therefore, increase the sensitivity to weak echoes generated from blood cells, a high-frequency transducer is often advantageous. However, at higher frequencies, the rate of attenuation of the sound beam by the intervening tissues becomes greater. Therefore, as with B-mode imaging, two opposing frequency-dependent effects (in the case of Doppler, penetration and scattered echo intensity) must be balanced by matching the transducer transmit frequency with the depth of the region of interest.

Doppler transducers usually operate in the frequency range of 2–10 MHz, because other constraints are placed on the system: a single transducer with dual imaging and Doppler functions, a desired frequency range for Doppler shift frequency, and the problem of aliasing (discussed later in this chapter). High transmit frequencies, typically 5–7 MHz, are employed for peripheral vascular Doppler examinations, whereas examinations of deep-seated vessels are performed at frequencies near 2 MHz. Most often, the transmitted Doppler frequency is somewhat lower than the nominal imaging frequency of the transducer. For example, a transducer labeled as "5 MHz" refers specifically to the B-mode imaging frequency. The transmitted frequency of sound used for Doppler evaluation in that same transducer will likely be in the range of 2–3 MHz. Some ultrasound instruments display the actual transmitted frequency used for Doppler, while others display only descriptors such as "resolution/penetration" while in the Doppler mode.

Doppler Display

Doppler units are designed to extract the Doppler shift frequencies from received signals. The Doppler shift frequency is in the audible range (typically between 200 and 15,000 Hz). Therefore, loudspeakers are used as output devices in addition to any other type of available display. Nearly all commercially available systems provide an audio display of the Doppler signal, as the human ear is extremely sensitive to Doppler signals. For visual display, the preferred format is to convert the measured Doppler shift frequency to velocity, which is independent of instrument parameters. Doppler displays utilizing frequency expressed in kilohertz, without velocity information, are not readily comparable when multiple examinations are performed by different sonographers on different instruments.

CONTINUOUS-WAVE DOPPLER

A continuous-wave (CW) Doppler transducer contains two piezoelectric elements: one to transmit the sound waves of constant frequency continuously and one to receive the echoes continuously (Figure 5-5). A single-element transducer cannot send and receive at the same time. Since the transmitted sound wave

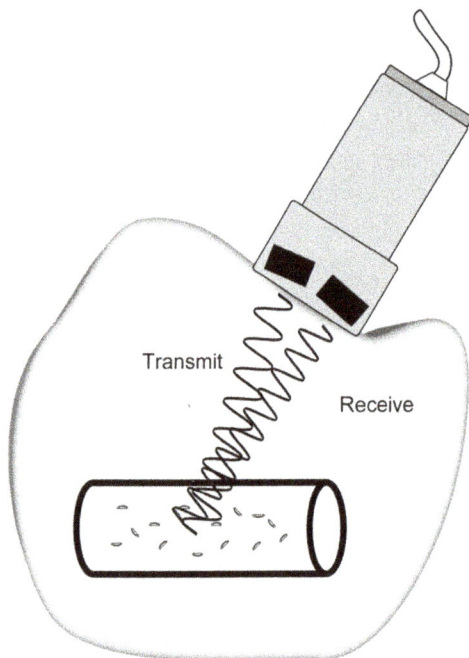

FIGURE 5-5. Continuous-wave Doppler transducer. Pencil-type probe has two piezoelectric crystals: one transmits continuously, the other receives continuously.

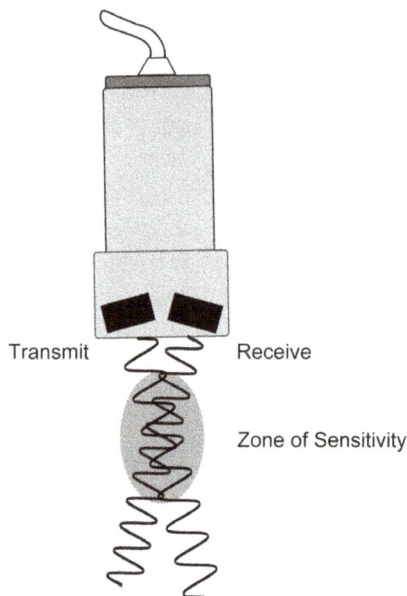

FIGURE 5-6. Zone of sensitivity for CW Doppler transducer.

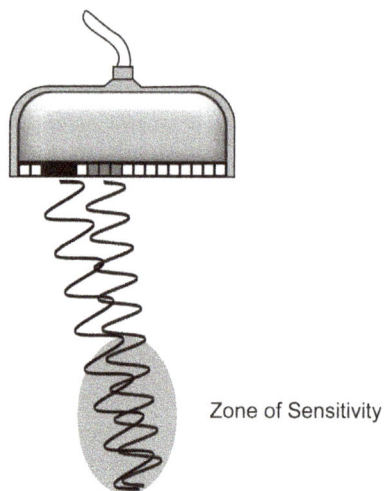

FIGURE 5-7. Multiple-element array transducer operating in CW Doppler mode. One group of elements (black) is designated for transmission and another group (gray) is assigned for reception. A zone of sensitivity is created where the wave patterns overlap.

is not pulsed, broad bandwidth transducers are not practical or even appropriate (wide frequency range yields multiple Doppler shifts for a reflector moving at constant velocity).

The sampling volume is restricted by the transmitted ultrasonic field (dependent on the frequency and focal properties of the sound beam) and the geometric arrangement of the elements. For the detection of a moving reflector located along the path of the transmitted beam, the resulting echo must strike the receiving crystal. The sensitive volume, or *zone of sensitivity*, is defined by the intersection of the transmitted ultrasound field and the reception zone. In essence then, each two-element transducer is focused to a particular depth (Figure 5-6). The two elements are tilted slightly to allow overlap between their respective fields of view (transmission and reception). A multiple-element array transducer creates a similar zone of sensitivity in CW Doppler mode by dedicating one group of elements as the transmitter and another group as the receiver (Figure 5-7).

Depending on the clinical application, the sonographer selects a CW transducer with the appropriate operating frequency and sensitive region. In a multiple-element array transducer, the operating frequency and depth of the sensitivity zone in CW Doppler mode may be adjustable, depending upon the instrument.

Doppler Measurement

The transmitted sound wave interacts with various reflectors, some of which are stationary and others moving. A fraction of the incident sound intensity is reflected at each interface. If the reflector is stationary, the frequency of the reflected sound wave is the same as the transmitted frequency, and consequently no change in frequency is observed. A moving interface causes the frequency of the echo to shift up or down depending on whether the movement is toward or away from the sound source.

Measurement of the Doppler shift frequency is based on the principle of wave interference. The Doppler effect causes the reflected wave received from a moving interface to vary slightly in frequency from the original transmitted wave. When waves with different frequencies are algebraically added together, they yield a slowly oscillating broad pattern of peaks and valleys, called the beat frequency (Figure 5-8). The beat frequency equals the difference in frequency between the two waves (transmitted and received) and thus corresponds to the Doppler shift frequency.

Figure 5-9 illustrates the steps required to generate the Doppler signal. The oscillator regulates the transmitter to emit a continuous sound wave of a single frequency. Alternating pressure on the receiving element by the returning echo is converted to an RF (radiofrequency) signal. The amplifier increases the echo-induced signal level. The reference waveform from the oscillator, which mimics the transmitted wave, is then combined with the received signal at the demodulator, generating complex resultant wave by means of wave interference. This resultant wave is then processed to remove the rapidly oscillating components; however, the slowly varying envelope corresponding to the beat frequency (dotted line in Figure 5-8C) is retained. Isolation of the beat frequency yields the Doppler signal, which has a frequency equal to the Doppler shift frequency.

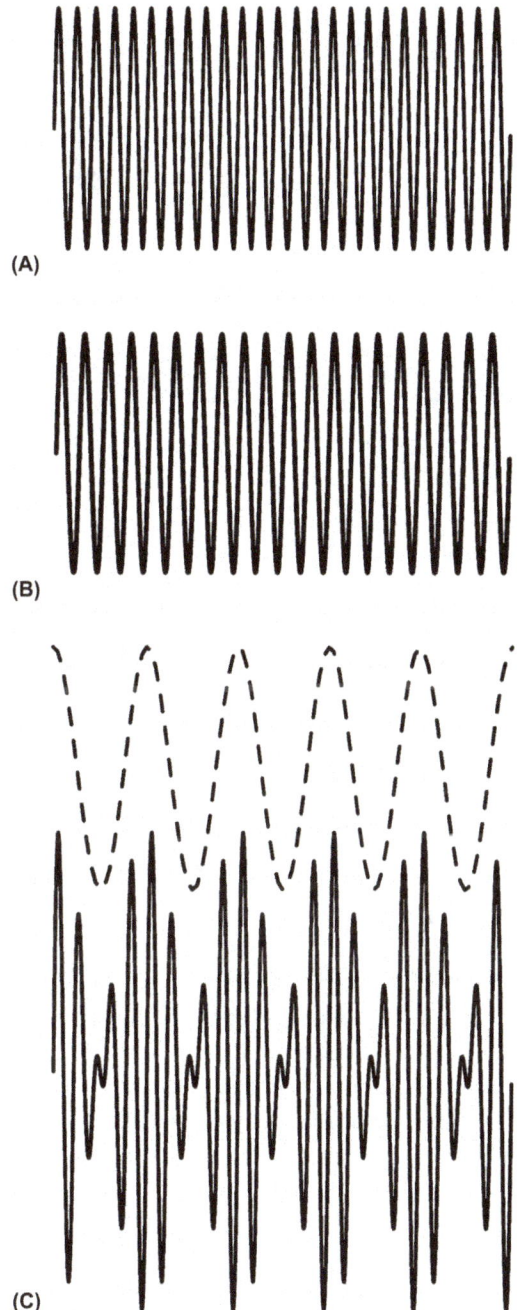

(A)

(B)

(C)

FIGURE 5-8. Doppler signal processing. (**A**) Continuous reference transmitted signal of constant frequency (25 cycles). (**B**) Continuous echo-induced signal of constant frequency (20 cycles). (**C**) Addition of the transmitted and received signals in A and B forms a complex waveform. The beat frequency of five cycles composes the outer envelope (dotted line) of this complex waveform.

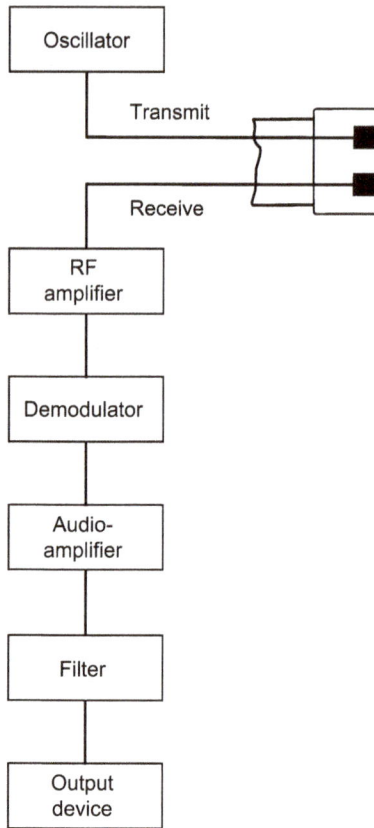

FIGURE 5-9. Schematic showing components of a continuous-wave Doppler unit.

Complex Doppler Signal

The signal processing illustrated by Figure 5-8 yielded a single-beat frequency, which denoted reflectors moving at a single, constant velocity. In a Doppler ultrasound examination of blood flow, RBCs within a vessel have a range of velocities that vary throughout the heart cycle and therefore, a range of Doppler shift frequencies will be present. The velocity of each moving reflector corresponds to a characteristic beat frequency upon echo detection and processing. Many beat frequencies representing all detected motion within the sampling volume comprise the Doppler signal. A complex Doppler signal is then formed by the summation of all the Doppler shift frequencies present after demodulation.

Signal Processing

The complex Doppler signal is amplified, filtered to remove unwanted low-frequency components caused by slow-moving structures such as vessel walls, and then routed to a loudspeaker for audible "display." The pitch of the audio output corresponds to the frequency shift between the transmitted and received sound waves and indicates the flow velocity within the vessel. As flow velocity becomes greater, a higher pitch is heard. A typical audio Doppler display for an artery exhibits a rhythmic rise and fall in the audible frequency due to the acceleration and deceleration of blood with systole and diastole.

Large, slow-moving specular reflectors in the body (e.g., vessel walls or heart valves) generate strong echoes with relatively low Doppler shift frequencies. These low frequencies produce a distracting thumping sound often referred to as "wall thump." Filtering removes these low frequencies, which are normally not of major interest and could mask other signals. The operator control, wall filter, rejects all frequencies below the threshold value, known as the cutoff frequency (Figure 5-10).

The cutoff frequency is usually set by default to remove Doppler shift frequencies below 100 Hz. Depending on the manufacturer and model, the cutoff

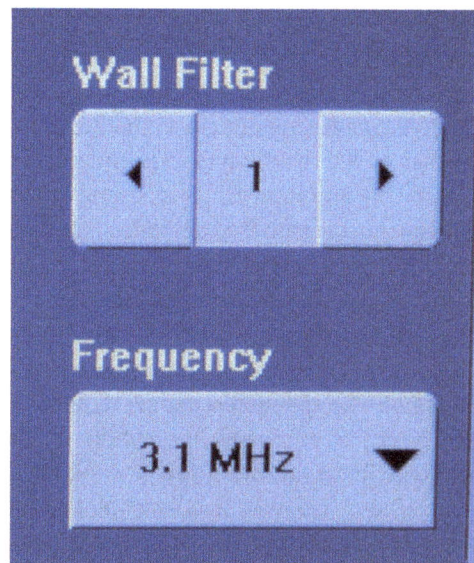

FIGURE 5-10. Wall filter control.

frequency can be adjusted to values as low as 40 Hz and as high as 1000 Hz (1 kHz). Most units automatically set the threshold value based on the study type selected in the preset menu. Because the wall filter control removes all frequencies below the cutoff value, care must be taken so that slow-moving flow is not excluded from the display. Thus, the wall filter should be set at the lowest possible value to remove wall thump while not eliminating any important blood-flow components of the Doppler signal. This is particularly true for slow venous flow as well as for the slight flow reversal that occurs in a normal triphasic arterial waveform (discussed in the following chapter).

Clinical Aspects

CW Doppler has high sensitivity to detect slow flow with low Doppler shift frequencies and, further, can discriminate small differences in flow velocity (Figure 5-11). The long sampling time of CW Doppler enables this modality to identify small changes in frequency corresponding to slow flow. At the other extreme, high-velocity flow is accurately measured with no limitation in velocity range. However, extensive flow volumes, such as those encountered within the left ventricle, cannot be accurately assessed with CW Doppler because precise depth information is not possible. The observed Doppler signal can be extremely complex, because the sum of Doppler shifts generated by all the moving interfaces within the sensitive volume is portrayed. If the sampling volume includes multiple vessels, the

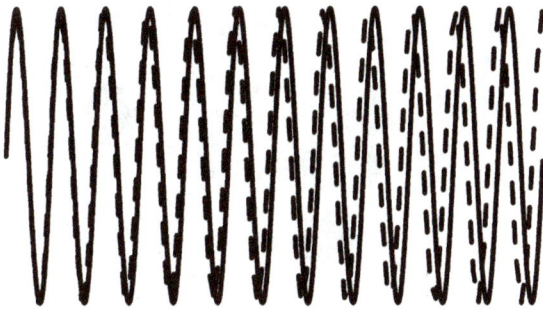

FIGURE 5-11. Sensitivity of continuous-wave Doppler to slow flow. The echo-induced signal from a slow-moving reflector (dotted line) requires several cycles to be differentiated from the reference transmitted signal (solid line).

superposition of resulting Doppler shifts becomes especially problematic. Therefore, CW Doppler is limited to those clinical applications in which sensitivity volume can be associated with a single vessel, such as the brachial or femoral artery. CW Doppler is commonly employed to evaluate flow patterns in heart valves. In this case, even though the large sampling area of CW Doppler records flow from other portions of the atria and ventricles, the easily recognizable flow pattern of the aortic and mitral valves is readily identified. Coupled with the fact that CW Doppler has essentially no practical limit to the velocity that can be measured, this modality is ideal to assess stenosis in valves, such as the aortic valve. (Aortic stenosis often produces velocities in the range of 500–600 cm/s, which would be impossible to determine accurately with a pulsed-wave (PW) Doppler system.)

PULSED-WAVE DOPPLER

PW Doppler provides quantitative depth information of the moving reflectors. Depth of echo formation is obtained via the echo-ranging principle in similar fashion to B-mode imaging. The transducer is electrically stimulated to produce a short burst of ultrasound and then is silent to listen for echoes before another pulsed wave is generated. Because of the requirement to assign depth, there is a physical limit to the number of Doppler pulses that can be transmitted in a given amount of time. Also, Doppler shift frequency determination entails longer pulse duration than in B-mode imaging. The necessity for increased pulse duration lies in the desire to detect received frequencies associated with slow flow that are almost the same as the transmitted frequency. Imagine that the pulse duration was confined to three cycles as in a typical B-mode acquisition (Figure 5-12). Certainly, the ability to distinguish small changes compared with the transmitted frequency becomes more difficult as pulse duration is shortened.

The received signals are electronically gated for processing so only the echoes that are detected in a narrow time interval after transmission, corresponding to a specific depth, contribute to the Doppler

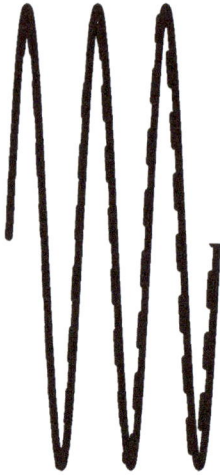

FIGURE 5-12. Pulsed-wave transmission of few cycles is unable to detect low-velocity reflector. Reference transmitted signal (solid line) and echo-induced signal (dotted line) are nearly identical.

signal. The delay time before the gate is turned on determines the depth of the sample volume; the amount of time the gate is activated establishes the axial length of the sample volume (Figure 5-13). Gate parameters are selected by the operator; thus, the

axial size of the sensitive volume and the depth of the sample can be adjusted. The axial sample length can be as small as 1 mm. The remaining dimensions of the sampling volume are dictated by the beam width in the in-plane direction and in elevation direction. Figure 5-14 illustrates the designation of the sampling region along the Doppler scan line in a B-mode image. Transducer frequency and focusing characteristics influence the dimensions of the ultrasonic field.

Multiple echoes from a moving reflector separated in time must be accrued to detect the motion. In order to achieve this, transmitted pulses are repeatedly directed along the same scan line to interrogate the sampling volume. Suppose a photographer took a single stop-action photograph (with an extremely short shutter time) of a car traveling west at 60 miles per hour. If you were shown that photograph, you would be unable to tell if the car was moving or not. And certainly, the direction of travel and speed would be indiscernible. However, if a series of stop-action photographs were acquired over a specific time period and then shown rapidly one after the other, the motion of the car would be clearly depicted, and the speed could be computed if the rate of sampling were known.

In PW Doppler, the basic CW design is modified to accommodate range gating and to collect successive processed echoes for analysis. Accurate time

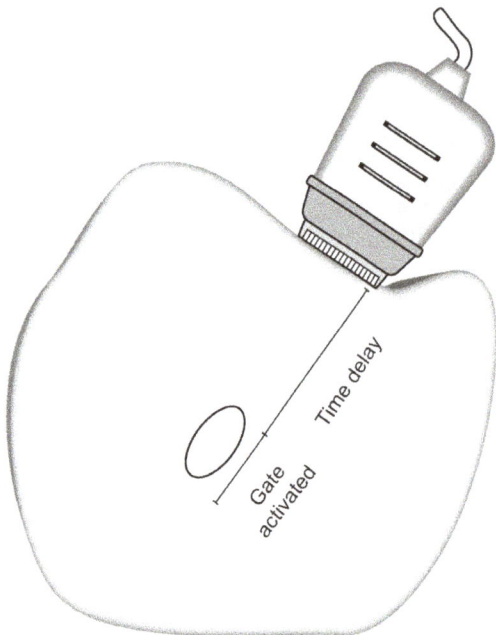

FIGURE 5-13. In pulsed-wave Doppler, the timing gate determines the depth and axial length of the sampling volume.

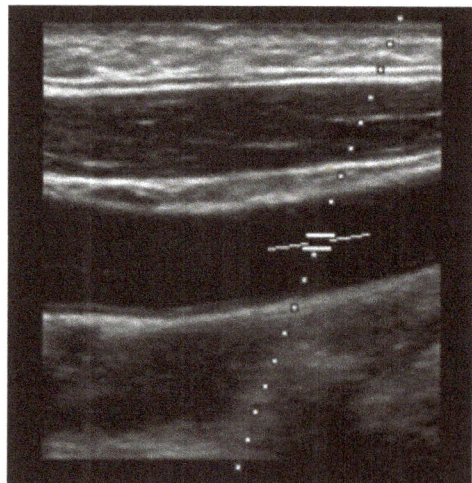

FIGURE 5-14. Operator-defined sampling area for pulsed-wave Doppler. The dotted line indicated the direction of sampling and parallel horizontal lines mark the axial extent of the sensitive region.

registration is critical for proper depth assignment of the Doppler signals. Gating is based on elapsed time following each transmitted pulse, and the time between consecutive echoes from a reflector is set by the pulse repetition period (PRP). The PRP is the time interval from the beginning of one transmit pulse to the beginning of the next transmit pulse. A single gate limits the interrogation to one depth along the scan line. The direction of sampling is indicated on the display by the Doppler cursor. Echoes formed along the Doppler scan line, but outside the sampling volume, are rejected. Only those echoes generated from within the sampled volume contribute to the Doppler display.

For reflectors moving at uniform and constant velocity within the sampling volume, a series of echoes from successive transmitted pulses are acquired over time. The depth-specific echo from each transmitted pulse, when processed, provides a single instantaneous value of the Doppler signal (beat frequency). The measured values obtained from multiple transmitted pulses are combined to form the time-varying contour of the Doppler shift frequency (Figure 5-15).

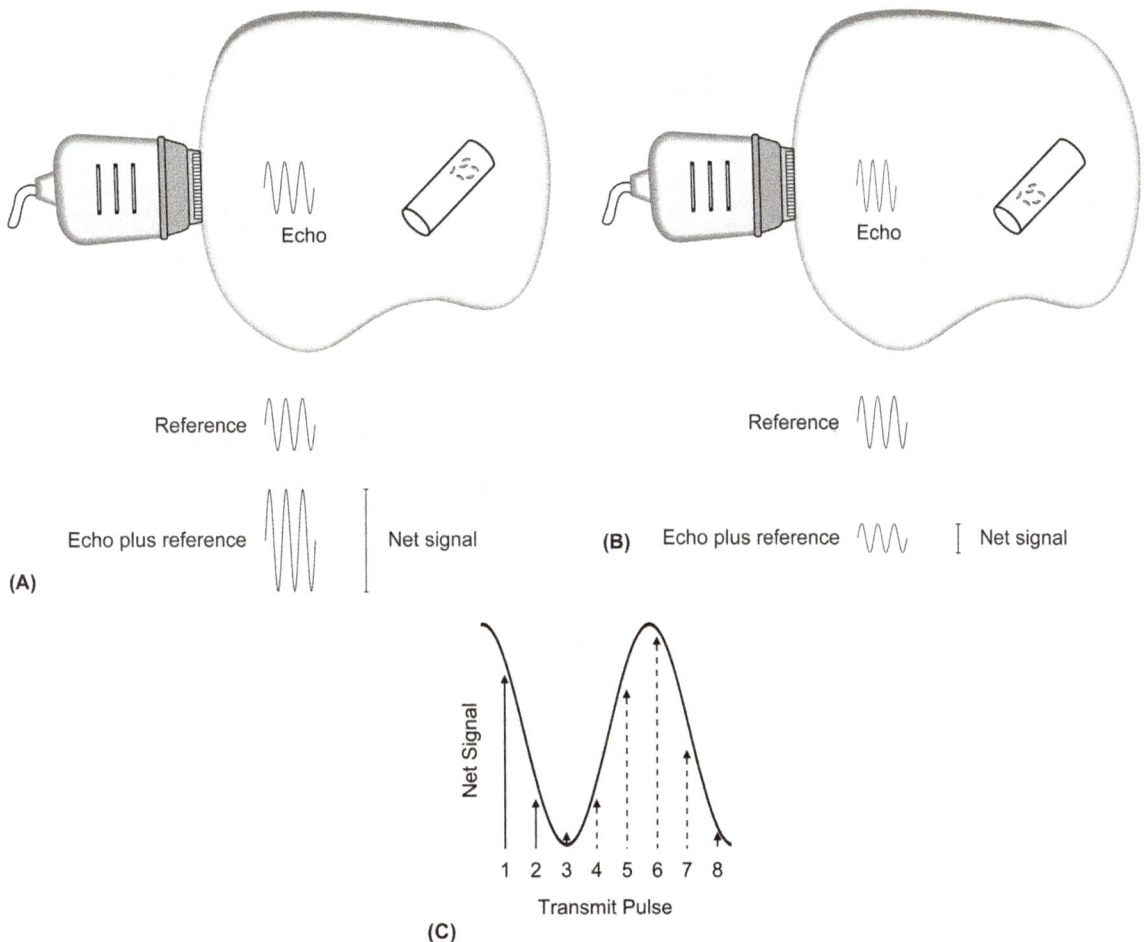

FIGURE 5-15. Pulsed-wave Doppler signal processing. A series of transmitted pulses are directed along the Doppler line of sight. (**A** and **B**) For each transmitted pulse, the echo-induced signal from moving reflectors within the sampling volume is combined with the reference signal to yield the net signal. The net signal from successive transmit pulses varies due reflector movement. Note the change in position of RBCs between transmit pulses in (A) and (B). (**C**) The net signals from multiple transmitted pulses when placed on a time axis compose the beat frequency. The first two points of sampling from A and B are shown as solid lines. Subsequent measurements are indicated by the dotted lines. Connecting all the data points yields the projected beat frequency.

In essence, the transmitted pulse rate (Doppler pulse repetition frequency or PRF) indicates how often the Doppler signal is sampled. Typically, a sequence of 64–128 pulses is transmitted along the line of sight to interrogate flow within the sample volume. The total observation time is usually 10 ms or less.

In PW Doppler, the beat frequency is not as well defined as with CW Doppler, because the pulsed echoes are equivalent to sampling the Doppler signal at discrete intervals. The oscillatory pattern can be more accurately delineated if the sampling occurs repeatedly at short intervals. This requires a high Doppler PRF.

Blood flows with a range of velocities within the sample volume and gives rise to multiple Doppler shift frequencies. These combine via interference to yield a complex Doppler signal, which represents all flow velocities present in the sampled volume. Fortunately, methods have been developed to isolate the individual velocity components and then display this information in an easy to understand format.

Velocity Detection Limit

PW Doppler has a limit with respect to the maximum beat frequency that can be detected accurately. This upper frequency boundary is called the Nyquist limit, which is caused by discrete (noncontinuous) sampling. The maximum Doppler shift frequency equals one-half the sampling rate, given by the Doppler PRF. Noncontinuous sampling creates a very important impediment in PW Doppler. To accurately measure a fast moving reflector producing a high Doppler shift frequency, a rapid sampling rate is necessary; however, a high PRF restricts the depth that can be interrogated, because a specific time is required to receive the echoes arising from that depth before the next transmitted pulse. Thus, as the depth to the vessel or structure is increased, more time is required between transmit pulses, and the maximum Doppler shift frequency that can be measured becomes lower. The problem becomes more complex because the Doppler shift frequency is also proportional to the transmitted frequency. The most problematic situation for PW Doppler occurs for deep-lying structures with high-velocity flow in which the Doppler angle to flow

is near 0 degrees. This combination of factors arises frequently in the Doppler evaluation of heart valves, particularly with disorders such as aortic stenosis in which the velocities can be very high.

Table 5-1 illustrates the effect of the depth of interest and transmitted frequency on the maximum velocity limit when angle to flow is unchanged. As the depth of interest is increased, the maximum reflector velocity that can be measured is decreased. Importantly, a low-frequency transducer allows higher velocities to be detected. A larger Doppler angle extends the maximum velocity limit. At a depth of 10 cm with 5 MHz transmitted frequency, the maximum velocity limit increases from 84 to 119 cm/s when the Doppler angle is changed from 45 to 60 degrees. This velocity constraint occurs because the motion of the reflector is sampled at discrete intervals and not continuously, as with CW Doppler ultrasound. In contrast with PW Doppler, CW Doppler has no maximum velocity limit. (Since the CW transducer is continuously transmitting, there is essentially no "pulse repetition frequency" and therefore no Nyquist limit).

The following is a real-world example which illustrates a practical application of the maximum velocity limit in a Doppler examination. The maximum PRF

TABLE 5-1 • Maximum Velocity Limit in Pulsed-Wave Doppler with Different Transmit Frequencies

Depth (cm)	Maximum Velocity Limit* (cm/s)		
	2 MHz	5 MHz	10 MHz
1	2096	838	419
5	419	168	84
10	210	84	42
15	140	56	28
20	105	42	21

*The Doppler angle is 45 degrees.

for a 10 cm depth is approximately 7700 pulses per second. Using a 3.5-MHz transducer with a Doppler angle of 30 degrees, the maximum Doppler shift frequency, which can be accurately measured, is 3850 Hz, or a velocity of 98 cm/s. If the transmit frequency were lowered to 2 MHz, the maximum detectable velocity would increase to 171 cm/s. Changing the depth of interest to 15 cm while maintaining the transducer frequency at 3.5 MHz reduces the detectable maximum velocity to 65 cm/s. Fortunately, these conditions are such that the physiologic velocities of *normal* velocity blood flow (except within the heart) usually occur within the detectable range of PW Doppler units.

Aliasing

At a minimum, two measurements are required per beat cycle to define the Doppler shift frequency unambiguously. This is the reason the Nyquist limit (upper limit for detection of the Doppler shift frequency) is equal to one-half the Doppler PRF. Because the beat frequency is sampled intermittently in PW Doppler, limited data are available for calculation of the Doppler shift (each transmit pulse ultimately contributes one point on the waveform of the Doppler shift frequency). If the Doppler PRF is not adequate to generate at least two points per beat cycle of the Doppler shift frequency, the Doppler shift frequencies above the Nyquist limit will be misinterpreted as lower than their actual value (Figure 5-16). This error in the measurement of the Doppler shift frequency caused by a low sampling rate is called aliasing.

Imagine that a race car is traveling around an oval racetrack at constant speed. A series of photographs closely spaced in time would accurately depict the motion as the car advances around the track. Indeed, as long as at least two photographs are taken for each lap, the interpretation of the movement would be correct. Now suppose the car accelerates to a higher speed, while the frequency of the photographs remains unchanged. At this faster speed,

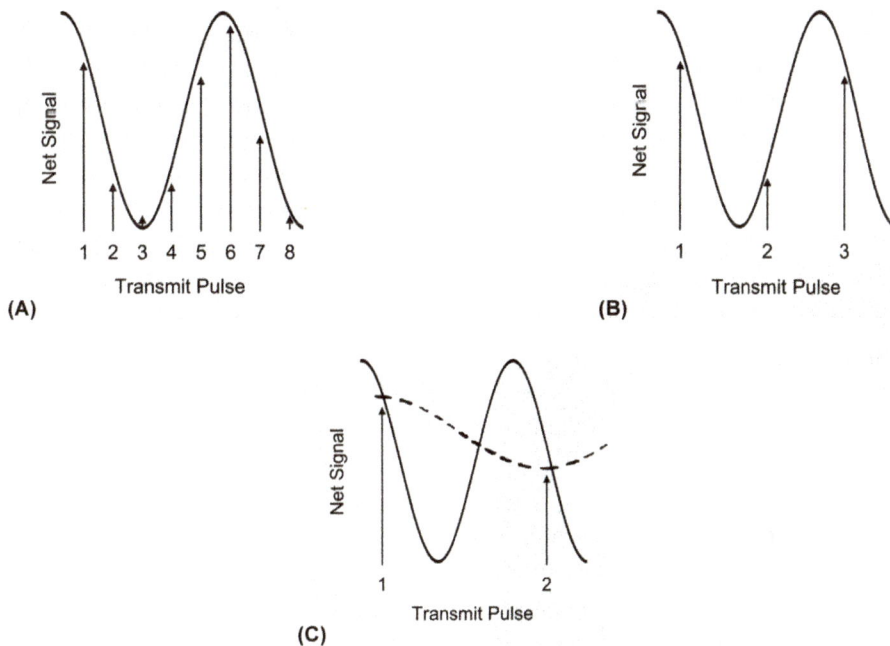

FIGURE 5-16. Intermittent sampling of the beat frequency (solid line). (**A**) Multiple measurements per cycle allow accurate assessment of the beat frequency. (**B**) As few as two measurements per cycle also provide accurate interpretation of the beat frequency. (**C**) If the sampling rate is less than two times per cycle, then the true beat frequency (solid line) is misinterpreted as a lower frequency (dotted line).

there may be 1.5 photographs taken for each lap of the car (three photos every two laps). This series of photographs will now appear to show the car moving backward around the track at slower than the actual speed. Thus, there is a *minimum sampling rate* (2 photos per lap) that accurately portrays the motion of the car around the track, analogous to the minimum sampling rate, or PRF, in Doppler applications.

Because velocity information is almost always displayed in velocity units as opposed to frequency units, the Nyquist limit is typically given in velocity. The Nyquist limit may be displayed separately from the velocity scale; however, it is important for the sonographer to know that the Nyquist limit is equal to the maximum velocity shown on the scale. There are both a positive and a negative value displayed for the Nyquist limit. If the baseline is moved up or down from the middle of the spectral display, the maximum velocity limit for forward and reverse flow is no longer the same (Figure 5-17).

If the baseline is moved all the way to the top or bottom of the spectral display, the Nyquist limit is extended to the greatest possible value in a single direction for the given sampling rate. However, any flow that is present in the opposite direction is unknown (Figure 5-18).

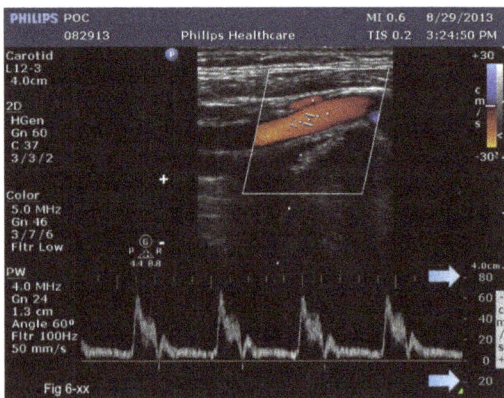

FIGURE 5-18. Baseline is moved to the bottom of the display. Measurements of velocity are restricted to one direction only, but the maximum velocity in the forward direction that can be displayed without aliasing is extended.

DUPLEX SCANNERS

Duplex Doppler units combine CW or PW Doppler detection with real-time imaging. The B-mode image depicts stationary reflectors (e.g., plaques inside the vessel and other anatomic structures), whereas the Doppler mode provides flow information within the designated region. The display of anatomic structures, such as vessel walls, aids in the selection of the sampling direction for both CW and PW Doppler and also in the placement of the sample volume for PW Doppler. Cursors showing these placements are superimposed on the real-time image (Figure 5-14). The Doppler angle to flow can be ascertained from the anatomy visualized on the B-mode image, and the sonographer must then adjust the "angle-correct" marker so that it is parallel to the anticipated direction of flow. This is most often accomplished within a vessel by aligning the angle-correct pointer so it is parallel to the vessel walls. The assessment of angle to flow in this case assumes that flow is parallel to the vessel wall (Figure 5-19).

While these assumptions may not be entirely correct, the errors introduced are generally small so that reasonable estimates of velocity are obtained. Visualization of the physical size and shape of plaque with real-time scanning aids in the diagnosis of vascular disease.

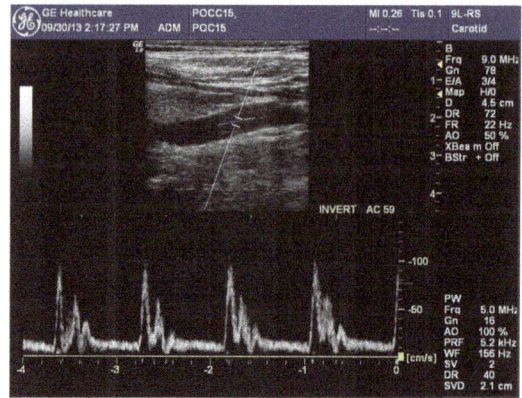

FIGURE 5-17. Baseline is placed off center. The maximum velocity in the forward and reverse directions is not the same (arrows). The + and − maximum velocity values are indicated by arrows.

(A)

(B)

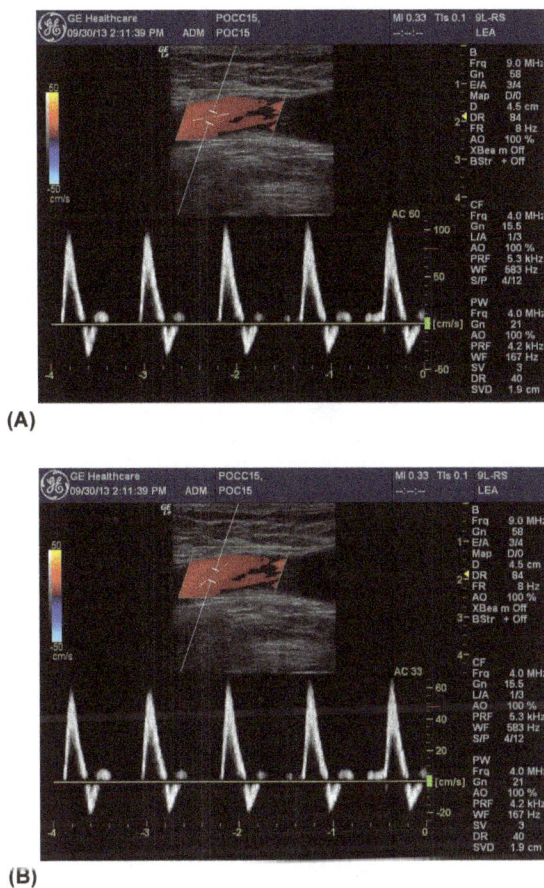

FIGURE 5-19. Angle to flow marker. (**A**) Proper angle to flow adjustment. (**B**) Incorrect angle to flow with resultant errors in displayed velocities.

The duplex scanner must perform both imaging and Doppler functions with near simultaneity. Because the optimal design specifications for each of these functions are not the same, various transducer configurations have been developed for the best combination of imaging and Doppler attributes for the selected clinical application. Current multiple-element array transducers enable the beam to be steered along the operator-designated Doppler sampling direction. In "simultaneous" duplex mode, real-time imaging is interrupted while the flow information is acquired, usually over a period of several milliseconds. The ultrasound beam must be repeatedly directed along one line of sight in the Doppler mode. A series of echoes from the same reflector arising from multiple transmit pulses is necessary to determine the beat frequency. The electronic interleaving of Doppler pulses between imaging pulses in duplex scanning permits real-time imaging, though at a reduced frame rate. In addition to reducing the real-time B-mode frame rate (degrading the temporal resolution), the simultaneous mode also lowers the available Doppler PRF, thereby creating a lower Nyquist limit for Doppler display. Doppler pulses must be given sufficient time to travel to the reflector and back, but, in addition, extra time must be committed between Doppler pulses to insert the B-mode pulse. For this reason, we recommend that the sonographer utilize the "simultaneous" mode for initial placement of the sample only, and then freeze the real-time B-mode image during active Doppler acquisition.

In duplex scanning, the flow information is acquired for a highly restricted region and displayed in real time. One of the major disadvantages of PW spectral Doppler in the evaluation of flow over a large area is that the global pattern of flow must be ascertained by sampling multiple, small regions one after the other throughout the field of view. This is very tedious, and isolated flow disturbances, such as small but significant stenotic or regurgitant jets, may go undetected or be underestimated.

A comparison between CW and PW Doppler modes is shown in Table 5-2. The characteristics of PW duplex scanning are presented in Table 5-3.

SPECTRAL ANALYSIS

If an artery is examined in cross section, it will be seen that RBCs at various distances from the center are moving at different velocities. Those closest to the vessel walls flow more slowly than those toward the center of the lumen. In a straight tube of approximately uniform diameter, the fastest flow velocities are in the center of the vessel. A sampling volume that includes a majority of the vessel lumen results in a Doppler signal that is a combination of many Doppler shift frequencies. Thus, the Doppler signal is a

TABLE 5-2 • Comparison of Doppler Instruments

Continuous-Wave Doppler	Pulsed-Wave Doppler
Cannot specify depth of sampling	Defined depth of sampling
Narrow bandwidth	Wide bandwidth
No velocity limit	Maximum velocity limit
High sensitivity to slow flow	Low sensitivity to slow flow
No aliasing	Aliasing
Real-time acquisition	Real-time acquisition
Measurement of flow velocity	Measurement of flow velocity
Range and distribution of flow components	Range and distribution of flow components

TABLE 5-3 • Duplex Scanning

Advantages	Disadvantages
Simultaneous display of B-mode image and spectral Doppler waveform	Small sample volume with PW Doppler
Ability to define sampling direction (and PW sampling volume) with respect to anatomy	Single line of sight with CW Doppler (all vessels along line of sight contribute to spectral Doppler waveform)
More accurate operator-defined angle to flow	No global presentation of flow
Measurement of flow velocity in cm/s	Reduced frame rates in B-mode
Range and distribution of flow velocities	
Real-time flow information	
Doppler and B-mode transmit pulses optimized independently	

complex representation of all the velocities present within the sampled region.

Spectral analysis is the process by which the complex Doppler signal is simplified into its individual frequency components. The relative importance of each Doppler shift frequency within the Doppler spectrum is also determined. This process would be comparable to listening to a symphony orchestra with the ability to identify the notes and number of each instrument that are being played at any given point in time. In this analogy, "sampling" the music repeatedly over time will result in different combinations of frequencies as well as type and number of instruments, as these factors change as the music is played. The mathematical algorithm used to accomplish this complex set of calculations is called fast Fourier transform, often abbreviated FFT. Fourier analysis separates the complex waveform into a series of single-frequency, sine waves. When algebraically combined, these single-frequency components yield the original complex Doppler waveform.

Figure 5-20 is a cross-sectional view of a vessel lumen. In regions 1, 2, and 3, RBCs move at different velocities through the vessel. The RBC's in region 3 are moving at the highest velocity, as they are within the center of the vessel lumen. Blood cells in region 1 are moving the slowest, since they are closest to

the vessel walls. For simplicity, assume that an equal number of cells travel through each region and the flow is continuous (constant velocity). If the Doppler sample volume is made very small so that each of these regions is probed individually, a characteristic Doppler shift frequency is obtained for each region (Figure 5-21). The Doppler shift frequency is highest for region 3, since blood cells in this region are moving at the greatest velocity. Because an equal number of RBCs are present within each region, and each region is sampled independently, the amplitudes (strengths) of the three Doppler shift frequencies are the same. Therefore, spectral analysis across the vessel shows that the heights of the individual waveforms are identical.

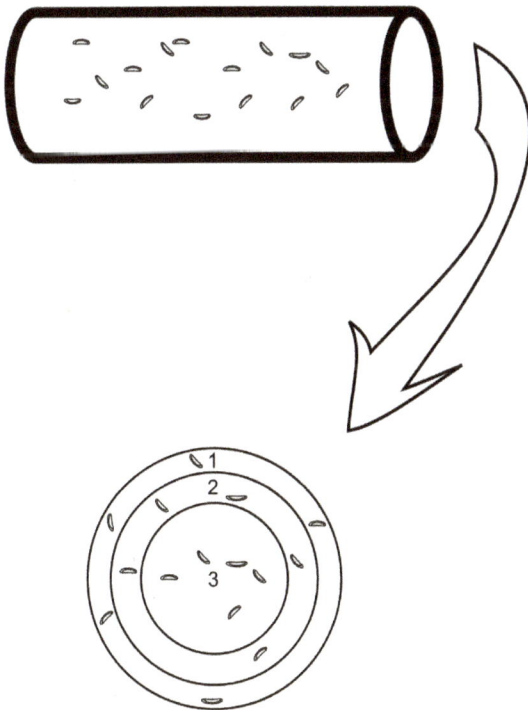

FIGURE 5-20. Cross-sectional view of three regions of blood flow across a vessel lumen. The regions 1, 2, and 3 are equal in size.

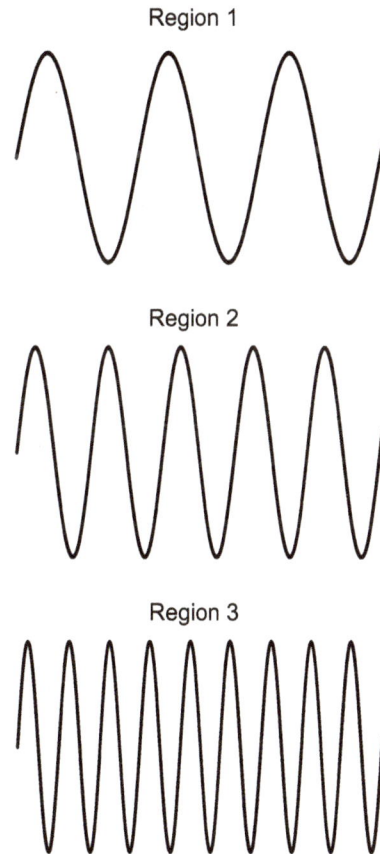

FIGURE 5-21. Doppler shift frequencies for regions 1, 2, and 3 in Figure 5-20. The Doppler shift frequency is the highest in region 3 where flow is the fastest and lowest in region 1 where the flow is the slowest.

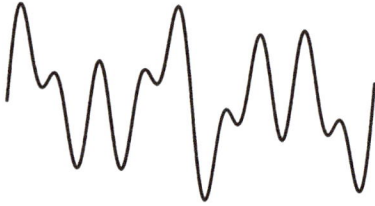

FIGURE 5-22. The sum of the Doppler shift frequencies in Figure 5-21 forms the complex Doppler signal.

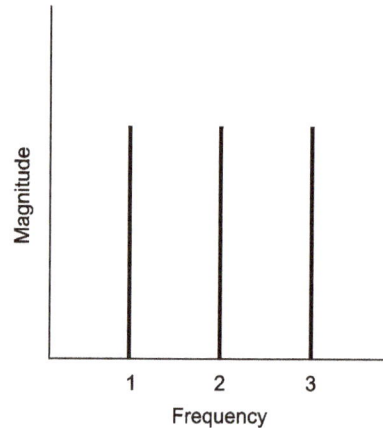

FIGURE 5-23. Power spectrum. Each flow velocity present in the complex Doppler signal in Figure 5-22 is depicted as a line. The three lines corresponding to the different regions of flow are the same height (same signal level).

If a longer axial gate is used, all three regions are sampled simultaneously by the ultrasound beam. Instead of three separate waveforms, each with its own distinct frequency as in the previous example, a complex Doppler signal is obtained, as shown in Figure 5-22. The complex Doppler signal contains all of the frequency components distributed across the vessel (in this example only the three individual waveforms in Figure 5-21 are present). The Doppler signal is then simplified by FFT to associate groups of RBCs with the corresponding Doppler shift frequencies (matching different flow velocities). With operator input of the direction of flow (defining Doppler angle), the flow velocity information can then be displayed in real time. Spectral analysis includes all of the individual velocities present at a given instant in time. Because the relative importance of each velocity is also determined, and thus, how "many" blood cells are flowing at each velocity, a comprehensive representation of blood flow at specific location along a given vessel or within the heart is achieved.

A power spectrum displays the magnitude of each individual frequency component plotted with respect to frequency. The power spectrum is an extremely useful analysis technique, because the desired flow information, the distribution of Doppler shift frequencies and the relative importance of each, is displayed directly. The magnitude is determined by the amplitude of the respective waveform corresponding to a particular frequency and represents the relative contribution of each frequency to the Doppler signal (i.e., the number of RBCs moving at the velocity given by the frequency shift). In Figure 5-23, the frequency components are shown

as three lines corresponding to the three velocity groups. The height for each observed frequency is the same since the initial assumption was that an equal number of RBCs is flowing through each region.

Suppose, for example, that the number of RBCs moving through region 1 is doubled. The amplitude of the beat frequency corresponding to this region also doubles and results in an altered complex Doppler signal. The Doppler shift frequency for region 1 remains the same, because the velocity of the RBCs has not changed. The spectral analysis presented by the power spectrum in Figure 5-24 depicts the increased importance of the lowest frequency by the increased height of the peak corresponding to this frequency. This type of display of the complex Doppler signal allows the sonographer readily to ascertain this increase in flow volume through region 1.

Now consider the power spectrum in Figure 5-25A in which the high-velocity group of RBCs produces twice the signal as the middle-velocity group, which in turn produces twice the signal as the low-velocity group. This information is converted to points of varying brightness (different shades of grey) along a straight line, representing the frequency axis (Figure 5-25B). Note that in this scheme of signal encoding, the high frequency dot is brighter than the middle

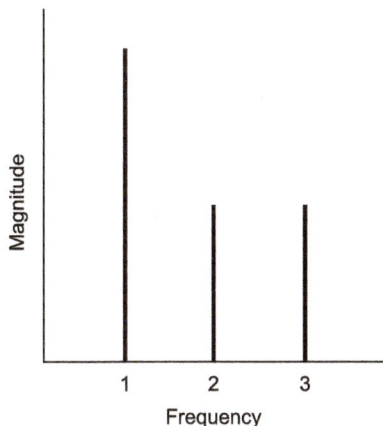

FIGURE 5-24. Power spectrum of the complex Doppler signal when the number of RBCs in region 1 doubles compared with those in regions 2 and 3. The flow velocity in each group is unchanged.

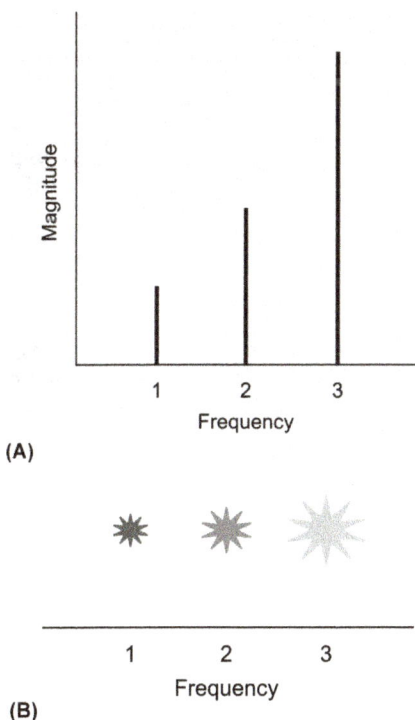

(A)

(B)

FIGURE 5-25. (**A**) Power spectrum depicting three discrete velocity groups in which the signal increases in importance from low frequency to high frequency. (**B**) Strength of signal for each group is converted to a bright dot. The brightness of the dot encodes the signal strength.

frequency dot, which is in turn brighter than the low frequency dot. In the spectral display, greater "numbers" of cells moving at a certain velocity result in that portion of the spectral waveform shown with a lighter shade of gray.

Thus, the on-screen spectral display has three components: Doppler shift frequency or velocity scale (vertical axis), time in seconds (horizontal axis), and magnitude of each velocity signal encoded by brightness level. At a given time when the power spectrum was acquired, each Doppler shift frequency or velocity detected is represented by a point plotted on the velocity scale with the brightness assigned based on the amplitude of the signal. Because the sampling and FFT analysis are performed in real time, sampling the Doppler signal repeatedly in small increments of a few milliseconds produces the time-varying Doppler spectral waveform (Figure 5-26). The time axis is typically displayed as scrolling across the screen (Figure 5-27).

MAXIMUM VELOCITY WAVEFORM

In vessels, the velocity distribution is not constant, but rather varies with time. Pressure differences in systole and diastole give rise to pulsatile flow within arteries. Venous flow is cyclical based on changing intra-abdominal and intra-thoracic pressure associated with respiration. Peak arterial flow velocities typically occur at peak systole. The peak, or maximal Doppler shift frequency corresponds to the fastest-moving RBCs within the sample volume at the time of measurement. Peak frequency (peak velocity) is an important descriptor of any arterial Doppler waveform. Arterial stenosis may often be quantified by measurement of peak frequency/velocity measured at specific location(s) along the vessel. The time-dependence of the peak velocity is depicted by connecting points of maximum velocity measured by the series of power spectrum segments. Most Doppler instruments have the capability to make this measurement automatically if the sonographer chooses to do so. This tracing is referred to as the

(A)

(B)

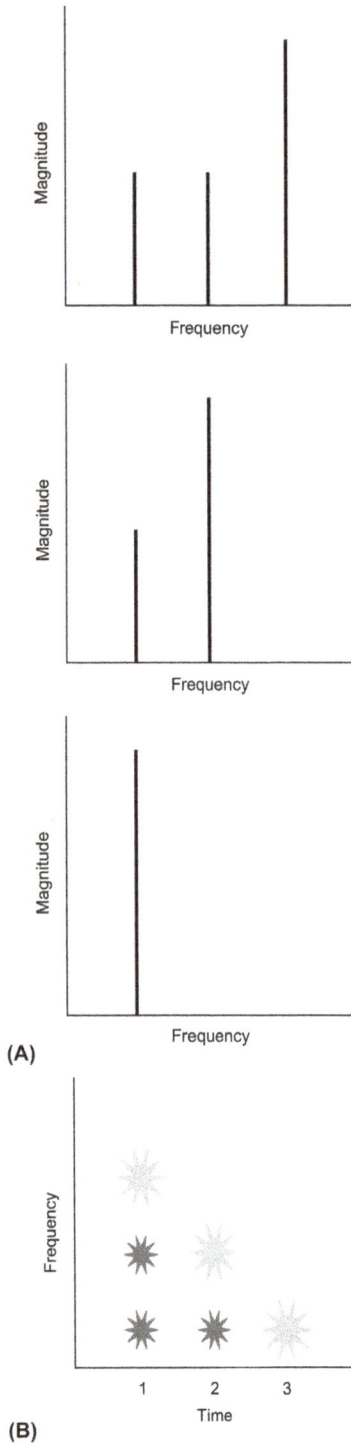

FIGURE 5-26. (**A**) Power spectra obtained by three measurements separated in time. (**B**) Time sequence of the brightness-modulated power spectra shown in A.

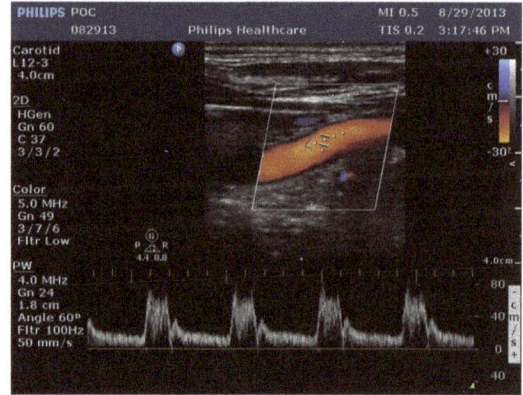

FIGURE 5-27. Doppler spectral waveform obtained for the carotid artery. The sample volume was positioned to encompass the central portion of the vessel.

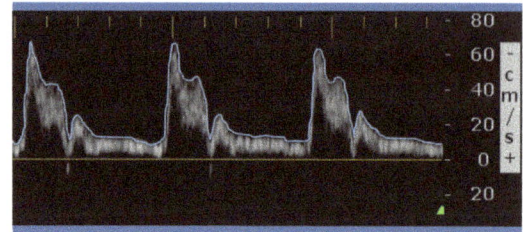

FIGURE 5-28. Maximum velocity waveform.

maximum velocity waveform (Figure 5-28). The maximum velocity waveform trace is also commonly referred to as the *envelope* of the spectral waveform. In addition to the peak velocity, the range and distribution of velocities present within the sample are also important indicators of the nature of flow within the vessel.

NARROW SPECTRAL WAVEFORM

In normal laminar flow within a straight artery of relatively uniform diameter, the distribution of velocities typically exhibits a fairly narrow range in the center of the vessel. That is, the highest velocity does not deviate very much from the lowest velocity during time of measurement. The spectral display, showing the magnitude of the Doppler signal at each velocity, contains a thin bright band which indicates that the majority of the blood cells are moving in the same direction, with only a slight difference in velocity. This type of flow pattern results in a *narrow band spectrum*, and is illustrated by the spectral waveform in Figure 5-29. Because the velocity distribution is limited to a narrow range, there is often an area "below" the waveform where very few bright data points are present. That is the case because virtually no blood cells are moving at those slower speeds. This creates a visible "empty space" under the curve of the waveform that is referred to as the *spectral window*, shown diagrammatically in Figure 5-29A and superimposed on an actual spectral waveform in Figure 5-29B. The presence or absence of the spectral window is an indicator of the nature of blood flow within the sample, and can be important in clinical assessment.

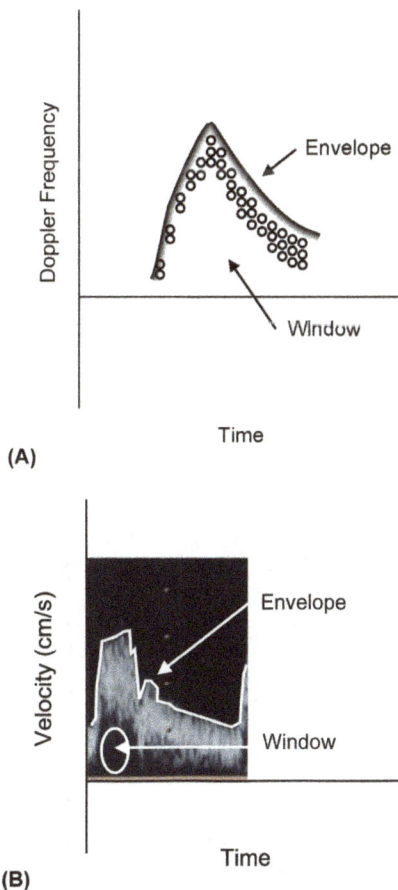

(A)

(B)

FIGURE 5-29. (**A**) Diagram of the Doppler spectral waveform. (**B**) Doppler spectral waveform showing the envelope and window.

BROAD SPECTRAL WAVEFORM

In the section above, patterns of blood flow in a smooth, straight artery were described. For vessels that curve, bifurcate, or change in diameter, laminar flow patterns become altered. The fastest velocities within a curved vessel usually occur nearest the outer or convex curvature. In this situation, eddy currents are often present within the lumen and exhibit small regions of retrograde flow. When a curved vessel is examined with PW spectral Doppler, a wide range of velocities will be present within the sampled volume. The increased range of velocity components are manifested on the spectral display as a "filling in" of the spectral window with additional bright data points representing slower velocities (Figure 5-30). Depending on the location of the sampled region, data points may be present below the baseline on the display, indicating that some blood cells are moving in the opposite direction.

PW SPECTRAL DOPPLER CONTROLS

The operator controls of velocity scale, spectral baseline, spectral invert, wall filter, sweep speed, power, gain, and audio volume enable the Doppler flow information to be optimally acquired and then displayed in

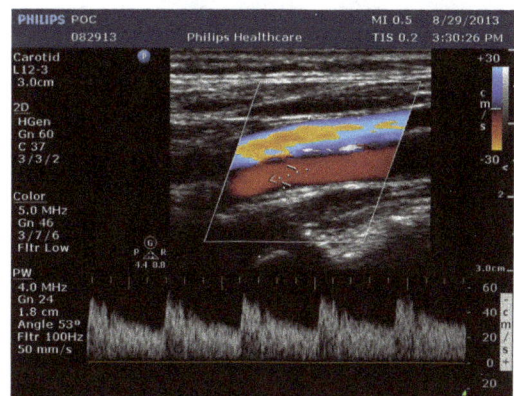

FIGURE 5-30. Broad Doppler spectral waveform showing loss of the spectral window.

a straightforward format. These PW Doppler controls are discussed individually in the following sections.

Velocity Scale

The spectral velocity scale control adjusts the Doppler PRF and is frequently referred to as the Doppler PRF control. If the operator wishes to increase or decrease the Doppler PRF, that may be accomplished by changing the velocity scale (Figure 5-31).

The PW spectral waveform is displayed as a scrolling trace where the horizontal axis is time in seconds and the vertical axis is the measured flow velocity (cm/s). As described previously, the amplitude of the various Doppler frequencies (velocities) is indicated by the brightness of the data points on the tracing. The spectral display is typically oriented so that flow toward the transducer is represented as positive (above the baseline) and flow away from the transducer as negative (below the baseline). The velocity scale should be optimized so the waveform is large enough to be evaluated easily, while remaining within the velocity scale limits without aliasing (fills approximately 75% of full scale as illustrated in Figure 5-32).

In PW spectral, Doppler aliasing is exemplified by "wraparound" from the velocity limit in one direction to the velocity limit in the reversed direction

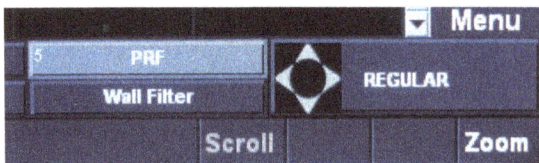

(A)

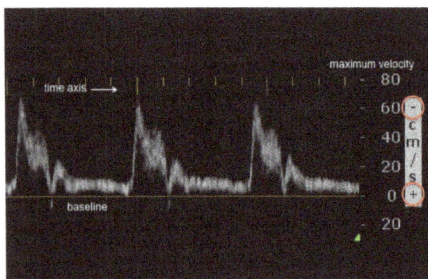

(B)

FIGURE 5-33. (**A**) Aliasing in which high-velocity flow is misrepresented at lower velocities below the baseline. (**B**) An increase in the velocity scale eliminates the aliasing artifact.

(Figure 5-33). Increasing the velocity scale may remove the aliasing artifact. Aliasing, along with strategies to reduce or eliminate it, is discussed in Chapter 7.

Spectral Baseline

The spectral baseline control raises and lowers the baseline, or zero-line, on the spectral display. Depending upon the type of examination and/or the preferences of the examiner, the baseline may be positioned in the exact middle of the display. Measurement of Doppler frequencies/velocities up to the Nyquist limit in both directions is possible. This is often preferred in cardiac applications, since bidirectional flow events are often seen within the same Doppler sampling area (Figure 5-34).

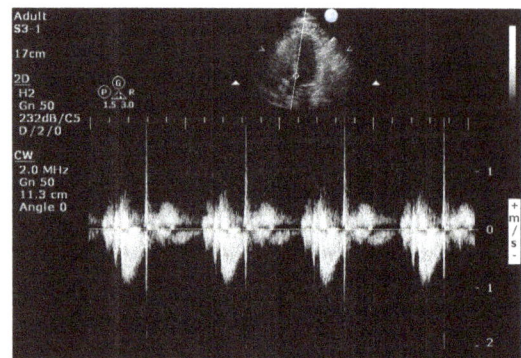

FIGURE 5-31. Doppler velocity scale control (labeled PRF).

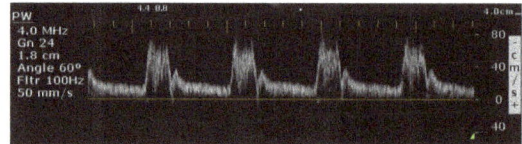

FIGURE 5-32. Spectral velocity scale showing + and – indicators (circled), baseline, maximum velocity, and time axis.

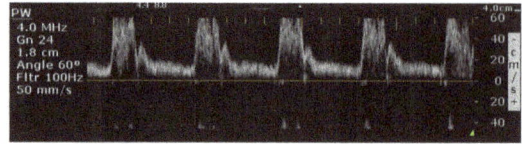

FIGURE 5-34. Duplex Doppler of aortic and left ventricular outflow waveforms. Baseline is positioned in the center.

In vascular applications, where a single vessel is being examined, equal distribution for both flow directions is unnecessary. Often, the baseline is placed about 1/4 of the way up from the bottom of the spectral display. This extends the Nyquist limit in the direction portrayed above the baseline, while still allowing some "room" for small negative flow events. This technique also allows for a larger image of the waveform to be displayed (Figure 5-32).

Spectral Invert

The spectral invert control establishes the direction of flow that is depicted above or below the spectral baseline (Figure 5-35). Depending upon the type of examination and/or the preferences of the examiner, certain waveform types may be preferentially displayed as "right-side-up," regardless of the actual direction of the flow in respect to the transducer. Vascular applications usually follow this preference. Note the (+) and (−) indicators along the vertical axis on Figure 5-32 spectral display. In other applications, such as echocardiography, the baseline is typically positioned in the exact middle of the display, and waveforms are portrayed in their "native" direction. That is, flow away from the transducer is always portrayed as below the baseline.

PW Wall Filter

The PW wall filter performs the same function as this control in CW Doppler. That is, all frequencies below the cutoff frequency (wall thump and low-velocity flow) are eliminated from the display. Figure 5-36

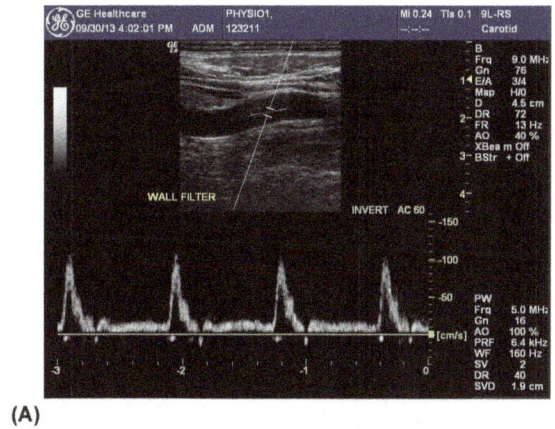

(A)

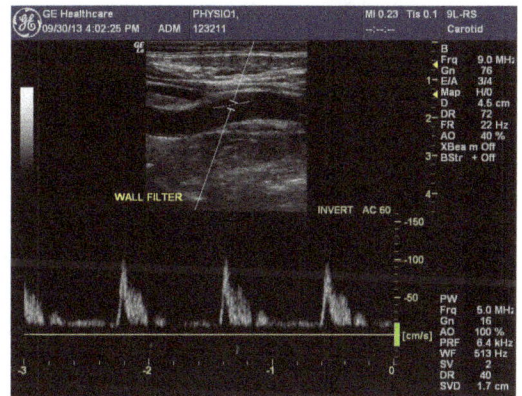

(B)

FIGURE 5-36. Loss of low-velocity components when the cutoff frequency is set too high. (**A**) Wall filter setting at 160 Hz. (**B**) Wall filter setting at 513 Hz.

illustrates clipping of negative component of external carotid artery waveform by selection of a high cutoff frequency.

Sweep Speed

The sweep speed is adjusted so that individual waveform features are spread wide enough to easily discern the shape. A sweep speed of at least 50 mm/s in usually required. However, a slower sweep speed such as 25–35 mm/s may be preferred when assessing the response of the blood flow to external maneuvers, such as limb compression or Valsalva maneuver during an extremity venous examination (Figure 5-37).

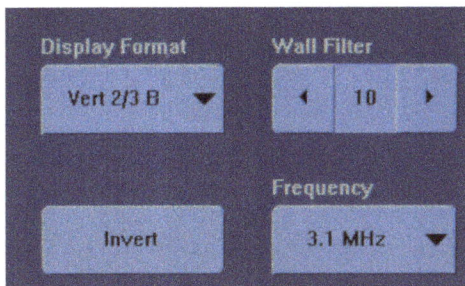

FIGURE 5-35. Spectral invert control.

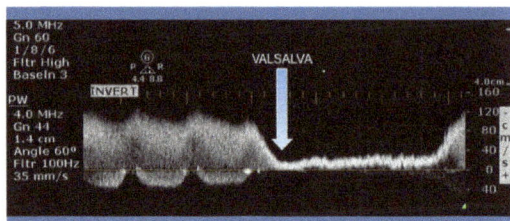

FIGURE 5-37. Duplex image of jugular venous flow with Valsalva maneuver.

Doppler Output Power

Doppler output power is set at a default value depending on the application preset selected. However, most units contain a power control enabling the sonographer to adjust the power level (Figure 5-38). Often, the Doppler output power can be reduced considerably and satisfactory results obtained by increasing the Doppler gain. The Doppler gain and Doppler output power controls are interdependent. Therefore, a decrease in output power must be compensated for by an increase in the overall gain. The control for the output power function may be several layers deep within the menu. For example, selection of the "more" or "page-2" soft key is required. Some systems utilize a Doppler gain/Doppler power toggle control. On many systems, the gain and output power control(s) are generically labeled, and function for whatever mode is currently active on the system. The output power control in both Doppler and B-mode varies the voltage to the transducer, and thereby regulates the amount of ultrasound energy delivered into the patient. On some point-of-care systems there is no direct control for the user to increase or decrease output power. In this case, the Doppler output power is adjusted automatically based on the exam preset and other parameters selected by the user.

Doppler Gain

Doppler gain is set at a default value depending on the application preset selected. As mentioned previously, a change in the Doppler output power requires a compensatory adjustment in Doppler gain. Doppler gain solely amplifies the echo-induced signal with no direct control on the amount of ultrasound energy transmitted. As in B-mode imaging, the sonographer should make adjustments where possible to set the output power at the lowest setting that provides the desired information. The general rule is the same as for B-mode output power: If a decrease in brightness is necessary, first reduce the output power and if an increase in brightness is necessary, first increase the gain.

Doppler Audio Volume

Doppler gain and the Doppler output power affect the Doppler audio output. An increase in either causes louder audio sound. The sonographer should be careful to not use the Doppler power or Doppler gain controls to adjust the audio volume. Doppler gain and output power should be set correctly first, then the audio volume should be optimized with the volume control (Figure 5-39).

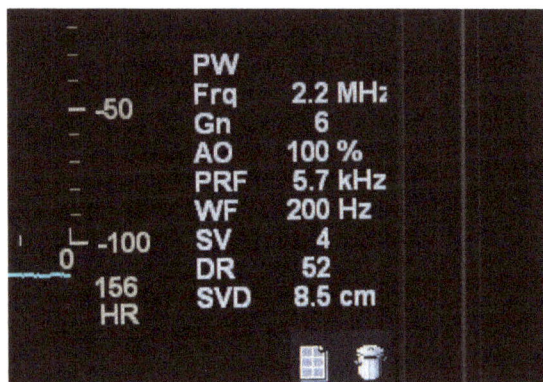

FIGURE 5-38. Screen display of Doppler output power setting (AO set at 100%).

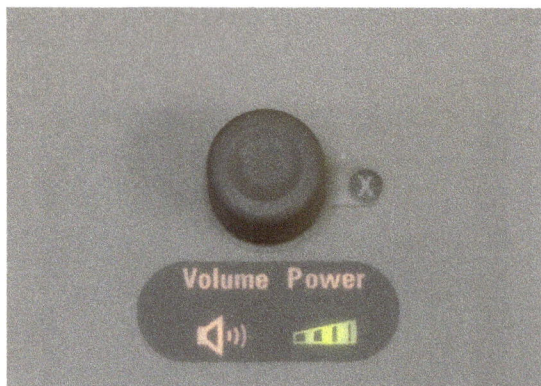

FIGURE 5-39. Volume control.

COLOR DOPPLER IMAGING

Although PW spectral Doppler has the advantage of providing a quantitative assessment of blood flow within the sampled volume, the information obtained does not easily translate into flow patterns over a large two-dimensional area. Color flow imaging, also called color Doppler, achieves that objective by visually superimposing Doppler information obtained over a large area together with B-mode information in real time. One transmit pulse per scan line is required to form the B-mode component of the color flow image. However, similar to PW spectral Doppler a series of transmit pulses are needed for each color scan line. The maximum frame rates in color flow imaging are slower than those achieved by real-time B-mode scanning. In addition to the time necessary for generation and reception of extra pulses, considerably more computational analysis is applied in color Doppler image processing. Even with these limitations, however, a frame rate of 10–20 frames per second is not uncommon. Motion is depicted throughout the scan plane by superimposing colors in various shades on the 2D gray-scale image. Color encoding in color flow imaging is based on a single parameter related to velocity.

Image Format

In color flow imaging, received echoes are analyzed with respect to signal level and frequency (Figure 5-40). Stationary structures, identified by the absence of a frequency shift in the returning echoes, are assigned a gray-scale brightness level based on signal strength as previously shown for B-mode scanners. Because moving reflectors cause a frequency shift in the received echo signals that indicates the presence and direction of motion toward or away from the transducer, the system assigns a color value to the pixel. *At each sampling site where motion is detected, a single representative velocity (usually the mean velocity) is color encoded. Colors are assigned a hue, saturation, or brightness, based on the measured velocity and the selected color map, and then superimposed on the gray-scale image.*

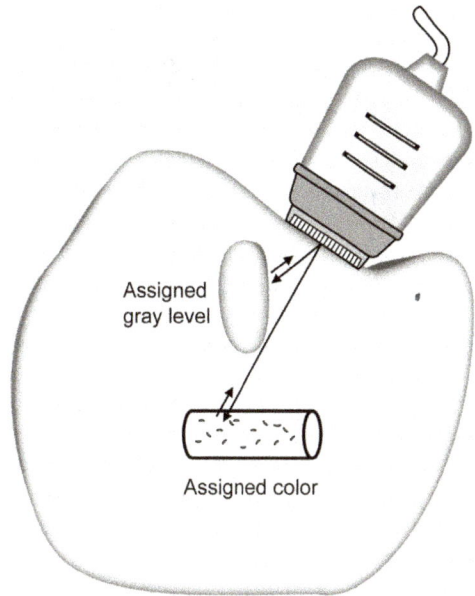

FIGURE 5-40. Doppler imaging. Echoes from stationary and moving reflectors are detected and processed to depict flow and anatomy.

Although the live real-time display gives the impression that color and gray-scale information are collected simultaneously, the color and B-mode scan lines actually are collected individually at different times. A color box defines a subdivision of the gray-scale field of view for color analysis. Color Doppler requires multiple pulses per color scan line (denoted by packet size), which directly impacts the frame rate. The color selection box or "color box" restricts the additional demands of color processing to that limited region, thereby improving overall performance and frame rate.

Color Assignment

A color map assigns various shades or brightness of color to depict different velocities while maintaining directional information (either toward or away from the transducer). The "red away, blue toward" (RABT), and "blue away, red toward" (BART) formats use color saturation to code for velocity. The lighter the shade of a color (more white added to the color), the faster the velocity. In the BART format, red indicates motion in one direction (toward the transducer), and blue denotes motion away from the transducer.

Fast-moving reflectors are represented in light shades of red or blue, and slow-moving reflectors in dark shades. The association of color with a particular direction of flow is interchangeable, however, and the color invert control allows the red/blue designation to be reversed by the sonographer. The sonographer must recognize that the assignment of color does not indicate arterial and venous flow, but rather the direction of flow with respect to the transducer.

Velocity Measurement

To accurately assess motion and assign velocity, multiple echoes from the same reflector must be collected using a series of transmitted pulses. Recall the analogy in which a series of stop-action photographs of a moving car allows its velocity to be determined, but a single photograph in the series does not indicate the presence of motion. Color flow imaging must determine positional information as well as velocity of the moving reflector. Spatial origin of the echoes along the Doppler scan line is obtained by the principle of echo ranging, in a similar fashion to B-mode. For each color scan line, multiple transmitted pulses contribute to Doppler signal formation. The color field of view is composed of numerous scan lines by electronic steering one series of transmit pulses after another along different sampling paths.

Velocity information must be obtained for a large number of sample volumes throughout the field of view in a very limited amount of time. The time constraint imposed by the requirement is that the image must be updated every 0.05–0.1 s (corresponding to a frame rate of 10–20 images per second). In addition, each image, or frame, consists of 100–200 scan lines. Range-gated, PW Doppler spectral detection with a dwell time of 10 ms for each scan line does not satisfy this condition, as fast Fourier analysis of each sampled area would take much too long.

Autocorrelation detection compares measurements acquired at each depth along the scan line using multiple transmit pulses. Processing of the echoes, segmented by depth to correspond with different reflectors, is done concurrently. For each transmitted pulse, the stream of signals from returning echoes along the entire scan line is placed into a buffer. Successive echo wavetrains are arranged on the same relative time scale, and thus reflector location is designated by the time interval following the transmitted pulse (echo ranging). The sampling interval along the scan line can be made 0.5 mm or smaller. At each segment assigned by depth, time-varying output from consecutive wavetrains indicates movement. Autocorrelation yields the mean velocity and signal strength for moving reflectors at each depth.

By characterizing the Doppler signal with a single parameter (usually the mean frequency), informational content (spectral distribution of the Doppler shift frequencies) is sacrificed, but the sampling time can be shortened considerably. Fewer transmitted pulses are applied along the scan line compared with PW spectral analysis. However, because of this, autocorrelation is less sensitive to slow flow and flow in small vessels. Therfore, care must be taken to adjust the color scale control downward if detection of slow flow is important (see more on color scale, below).

Typically, each scan line is sampled 4–10 times, although as many as 32 transmit pulses may be used. Packet size or *ensemble length* describes the number of pulses that interrogate a single color scan line. A large packet size (long integration time) provides the highest color definition (most accurate frequency estimates), but lowers the frame rate. A smaller packet size (fewer pulses) shortens the time requirement, but at the cost of somewhat less accurate frequency determination. Packet size is frequently adjustable by the operator, and decreasing this control is one way that the sonographer can improve the color frame rate (Figure 5-41). The sonographer must determine whether the velocity accuracy is adversely affected by the shorter sampling time. Many scanners automatically adjust packet size and color line density as a function of field width to optimize the frame rate for a particular application. The sonographer is then free to fine tune these controls manually if that capability is available on the system.

Image Acquisition

The gray-scale scanning is accomplished by generating sequential, dynamically focused beams along

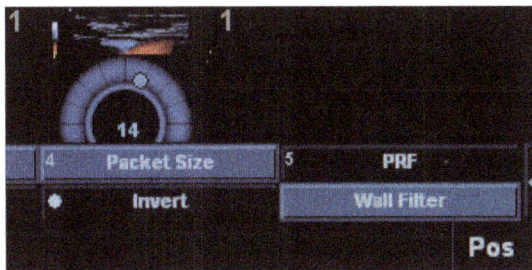

FIGURE 5-41. Packet size control.

the physical extent of a linear array transducer. Parallel scan lines compose the gray-scale component, which provides sampling perpendicular to the blood movement (the vessel is assumed to be parallel to the skin surface). Perpendicular incidence of the beam is desirable for imaging but not for assessing flow as the interrogation angle would be 90 degrees. To achieve a more favorable Doppler angle to flow, the beam for flow measurements must be steered at an angle to the array (Figure 5-42). Doppler angle to flow may be enhanced by utilizing a "heel-toe" motion of the transducer, as further described in Chapter 9.

If the beam is steered, the signal generated from returning echoes is directed to the Doppler channel. For non-steered beams, signals are directed to the gray-scale channel. The image data are processed

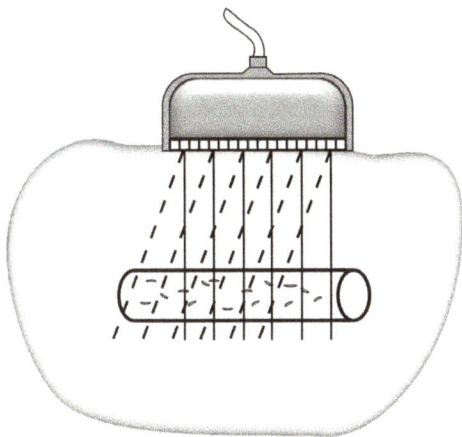

FIGURE 5-42. Color flow imaging with a linear array in which the gray-scale scan lines (solid) and steered color scan lines (dotted) are acquired independently.

and sent to the scan converter. In the Doppler channel, autocorrelation is employed to quantify forward and reverse flow signals. These are then numerically encoded and sent to the scan converter. The numerical values in the scan converter are translated into separate gray and color levels before the composite image is displayed on the monitor.

Because the acquisition is asynchronous, the autocorrelation scanner allows the transmitted beam to be optimized specifically for both Doppler and gray scale. The transmitted frequency, focal properties, and transmit power are adjusted separately for each mode of operation. Typically, transmission for color Doppler is at a somewhat lower frequency than that of B-mode. Doppler transmitted power may be increased to improve detection of weak flow signals. In order to optimize overall frame rate, low color scan line density, reduced color field of view, small packet size, or a combination of these may be used. Interpolation of color data fills in the gaps between color scan lines. The Doppler and gray-scale spatial resolution are not necessarily equivalent. Indeed, the axial sampling interval for Doppler is usually greater (as much as several millimeters). Since non-continuous sampling is inherent in color flow imaging, this modality is also subject to aliasing artifacts (high-velocity components are depicted with colors representing lower velocities). The characteristics of color flow imaging are summarized in Table 5-4.

COMBINED DOPPLER MODE

In the color flow image, a single parameter, usually the mean velocity represented by the variation in color, is spatially registered in two dimensions. PW spectral Doppler provides a more detailed presentation of the distribution of the velocity profile at a point of interest. The combined Doppler mode displays the color flow image with Doppler spectral waveform (Figure 5-43). A specific sampling volume for spectral analysis is identified by superimposing a cursor line with range gate on the color flow image. Since data collection is now shared between gray scale, color Doppler, and PW Doppler, the refresh

TABLE 5-4 • Characteristics of Color Flow Imaging

Advantages	Disadvantages
Two-dimensional display of global blood flow	Mean velocity only, no spectral analysis
Real-time depiction of flow throughout field of view	Limited frame rate
Guides placement of pulsed-wave sampling volume	Color aliasing
Regions of abnormal flow more rapidly identified	Motion artifacts
	Accuracy of velocity limited by sampling time
	Low-density color scan lines or limited color field of view
	Poor lumen definition
	Qualitative flow observations
	Doppler angle dependent
	Color artifacts
	Insensitivity to low-volume flow

rate of the color flow image is slowed to a new frame every 1–5 s. Areas with abnormal flow patterns can be rapidly identified, reducing examination time by facilitating placement of the sampling volume for spectral analysis.

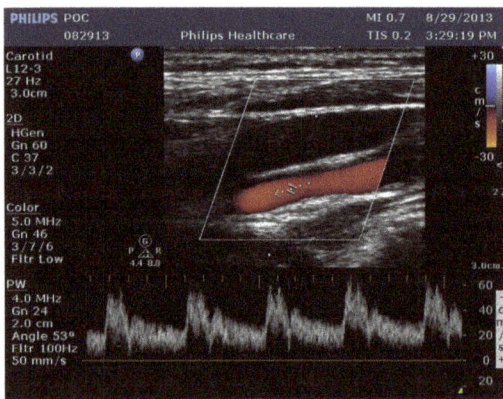

FIGURE 5-43. Combined Doppler. The sampling volume superimposed on the color flow image is defined for the Doppler spectral analysis.

COLOR DOPPLER CONTROLS

The operator controls of color box, color box steering, color velocity scale, color baseline, color map, color map invert, color wall filter, color gain, packet size, color line density, color transmit frequency, and color persistence regulate the acquisition and display of color Doppler information. These color Doppler controls are discussed individually in the following sections. Many of these controls have similar functions to those in PW Doppler.

Color Box or Color ROI

The color box or color ROI (region of interest) is displayed on the screen simultaneously with the B-mode image. Color analysis is only performed within the region defined by the box. Individual scan lines that include a portion of the color box require additional pulses for both color Doppler and B-mode analysis. Because increasing the size of the box can greatly reduce the temporal resolution by reducing the frame rate, the sonographer should limit the color box size to the specific area of interest. Color box size and position are usually adjusted by a toggle-type control on the console. Touching the control alternates between color box size and color box position. The size adjustment or box placement is then made utilizing the system trackball or trackpad. If PW spectral Doppler mode is also active, the control usually becomes a three-way toggle between color box size, position, and position of the PW sample.

Color Box Steering

Linear array transducers permit steering of the color box to the left or right (or straight down) on the B-mode image (Figure 5-44). This greatly facilitates achieving an optimum color angle to flow by the sonographer. Some systems allow fully variable color box steering, while other systems are restricted to three settings such as angle left, straight down, and angle right. Both systems still rely on transducer manipulation by the sonographer to achieve the optimum color angle to flow and the three-position system does not appear to have any significant disadvantage over the fully variable system in actual practice. Indeed, the curvilinear array and sector transducer systems do not allow color box steering at all, but instead rely completely on sonographer manipulation of the transducer to achieve an adequate color angle to flow.

Color Velocity Scale

The color velocity scale is incorporated into the color flow display and is shown as the color scale bar with the color Nyquist limit (maximum velocity that can be measured without aliasing) indicated. In color flow imaging, the color-encoded velocity is typically *mean velocity* and is most often specified in units of cm/s. Velocities less than the maximum velocity are portrayed accurately without color aliasing. The velocity range is set by the sonographer depending on the clinical application. Increasing the velocity scale enhances the ability to display fast-moving reflectors, while decreasing the velocity scale improves the partition of slower flow. The color velocity scale also controls the color PRF and is therefore frequently referred to as the "color PRF" control. At least one unit used this label on the control itself. The onscreen velocity color scale is usually referred to as the "color bar" (Figure 5-45).

Color Baseline

The color baseline setting is incorporated into the color velocity scale, and is denoted as a black, horizontal line on the color bar, separating the forward

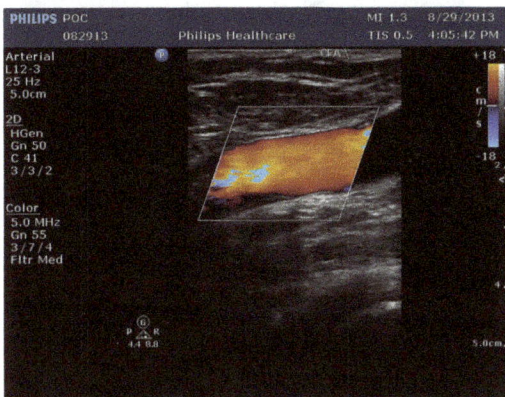

FIGURE 5-44. Color flow Image with an angled color box.

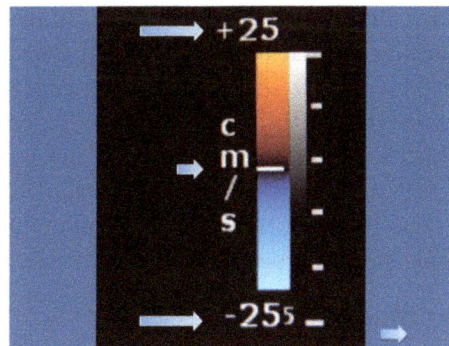

FIGURE 5-45. Color velocity scale ("color bar") with arrows showing color scale units (short arrow) and Nyquist limits (long arrows). Note the BART (Blue Away Red Toward) orientation of the display.

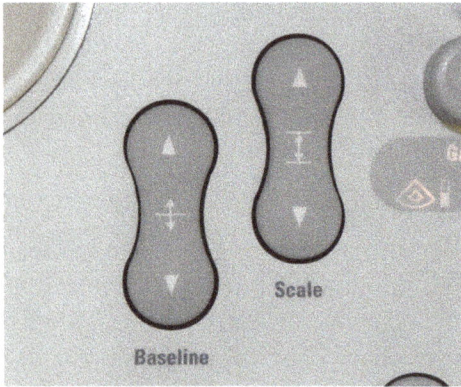

FIGURE 5-46. Color baseline control.

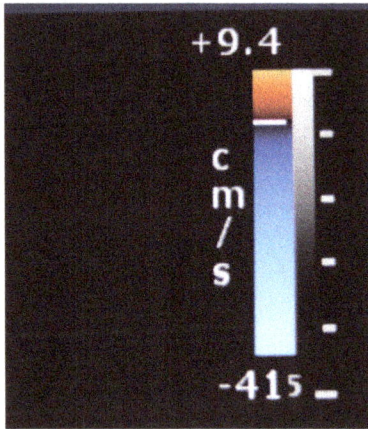

FIGURE 5-47. Color bar with an off-center baseline.

and reverse flow. The color bar is typically positioned in the middle of the velocity scale by default. However, the color baseline control allows the user to adjust the baseline from the midpoint toward the positive or negative side (Figures 5-46 and 5-47). This is sometimes helpful in order to accommodate higher velocities in one direction and is often employed to minimize color aliasing of high-velocity flow. (The ability to accurately display flow in the opposite direction is sacrificed.)

Color Map

In color flow imaging, numerous color maps are available to depict the range of flow velocities as different colors. Compare color flow images of the liver, in which four different color maps were chosen for the same scan plane (Figure 5-48A–D).

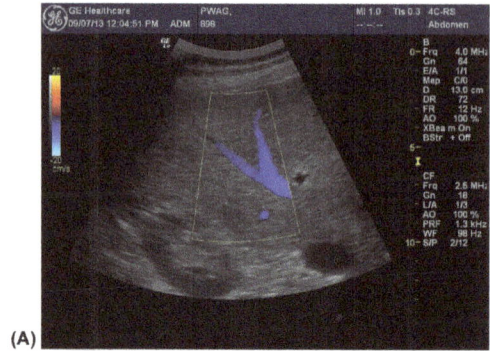

(A)

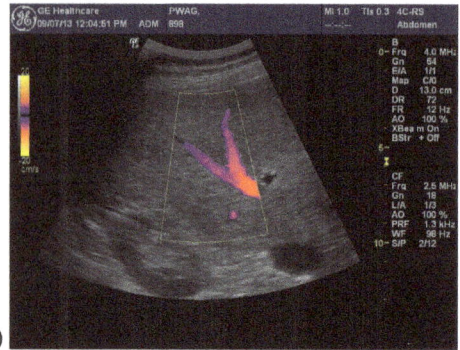

(B)

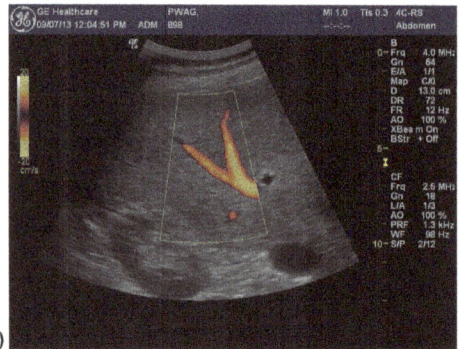

(C)

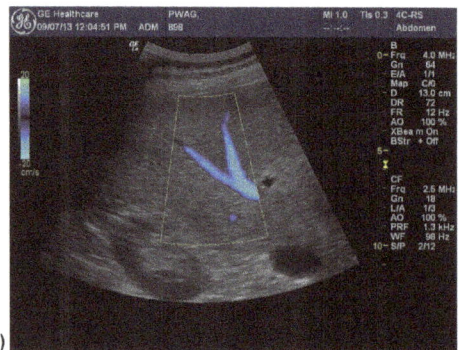

(D)

FIGURE 5-48. Examples of 4 color maps for hepatic venous flow. (A) Map 1, (B) Map 2, (C) Map 3, (D) Map 4.

The information content is the same, although the translation from velocity to color follows a different algorithm for each color map. Color map selection is based solely on operator preference. Typically, the sonographer chooses on color map setting which he/she likes, and rarely touches the control after that. Often, the default color map in the application preset is used without any changes.

Color Map Invert

The color map invert control allows the association of colors (e.g., red and blue) with a specific flow direction. This technique is most often utilized to permit arterial flow to be designated as red and venous flow as blue, regardless as to whether the flow is toward or away from the transducer. The assignment of color in this manner is somewhat controversial and is done according to personal preference, or preference of the lab supervisor. This choice of color designation is only practical when the examined vessel(s) are relatively straight. Flow within a twisting or curving vessel will alternately be oriented toward and away from the transducer and thus will be depicted as both red and blue, regardless of whether the vessel is a vein or artery (Figure 5-49).

Color Wall Filter

The color wall filter functions in the same way as the wall filter in spectral Doppler (Figure 5-50). As

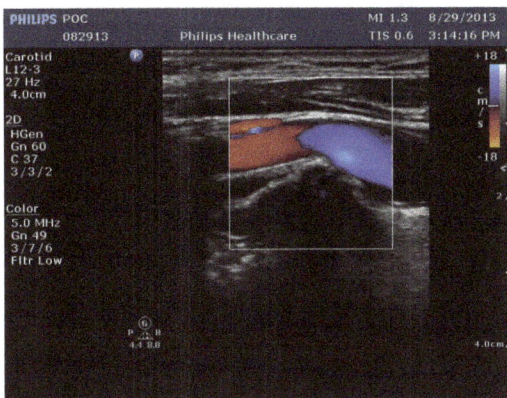

FIGURE 5-50. Color wall filter control.

the control setting is increased, lower Doppler frequencies (velocities) are eliminated from the display. The color wall filter can be helpful, if used in moderation, to eliminate extraneous colors caused by vessel wall motion. Typically, the default setting of this control for the particular application preset is adequate for that purpose. However, the color wall filter control is available on most mid- to upper-level portable systems and can be manually increased or decreased from the default value where necessary. Care must be taken to not set the control so high that actual flow information is eliminated (Figure 5-51). Too low a wall filter setting introduces extraneous color from wall motion (Figure 5-52).

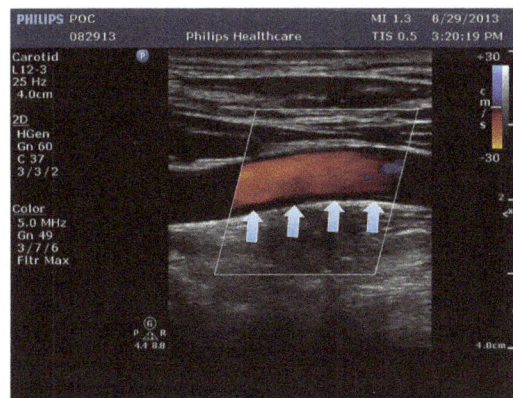

FIGURE 5-49. Color image of carotid bulb/bifurcation showing red and blue within the same vessel. Note the color map setting of RABT.

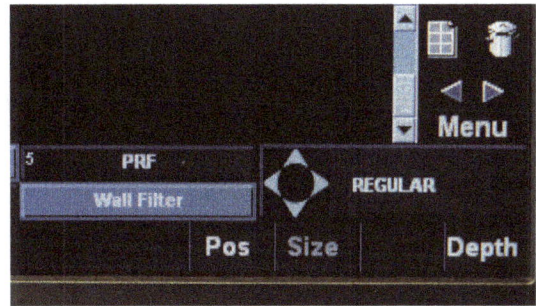

FIGURE 5-51. Color flow image with too high wall filter causing a loss of slow flow components along vessel walls (arrows).

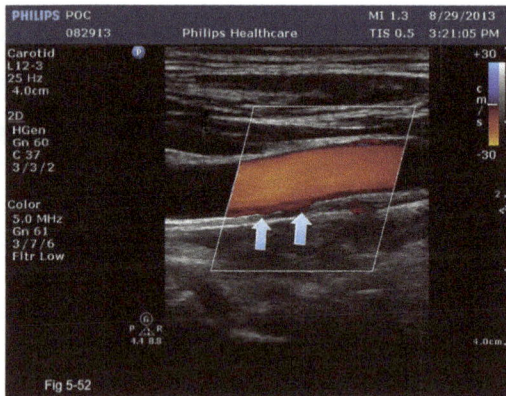

FIGURE 5-52. Color flow image with too low wall filter producing a wall motion artifact.

Color Gain

The color gain control allows the sonographer to adjust the amount of amplification of the color Doppler signal. Higher color gain increases the brightness of the color displayed on the screen. Color gain works in tandem with the color output power control (if available on the system). A decrease in color output power requires a corresponding increase in the color gain in order to maintain the optimal color brightness on the display. Color gain and color output power also modify the amount of "color filling" seen within the vessel or heart chamber. On systems without a user-adjustable color output power control, the output power is regulated by the system according to the selected examination type. If the expected amount of color does not appear within the examined vessel, the color scale setting may require adjustment to include either faster or slower flow velocities. Once the correct color scale setting is established, the color output power control (if available) and the color gain control should be adjusted to optimize the color display. Too low a setting of color gain results in incomplete "filling" of a vessel where flow is expected. Too high a setting causes "color bleed" outside the vessels walls into the surrounding tissues (Figure 5-53).

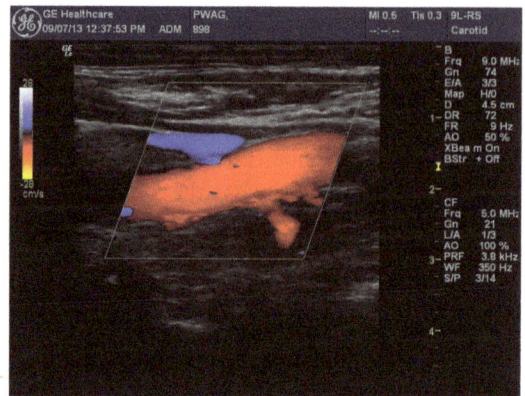

(A)

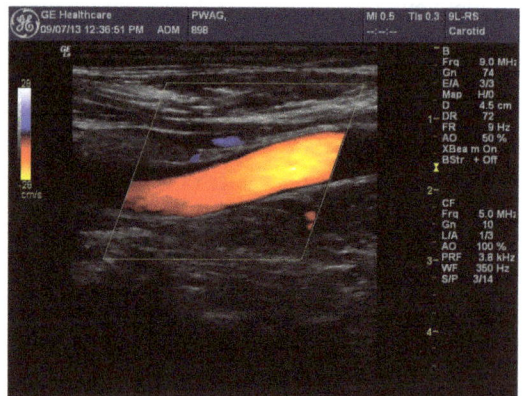

(B)

FIGURE 5-53. Color gain. **(A)** Color gain set too high. **(B)** Color gain set correctly.

Color Packet Size

The color packet size control varies the number of "color transmit pulses" employed to acquire a single color scan line (Figure 5-54). Color packet size is also referred to as ensemble length, and is adjustable by the operator on some instruments. As with other B-mode, color, and Doppler parameters, color packet size is set by default depending on the transducer and examination type selected by the sonographer. If the control is available, the sonographer may attempt to improve temporal resolution (color frame rate, in this case) by decreasing the packet size. The sonographer should be aware that a small packet size results in less accurate assessment of color Doppler frequencies/velocities.

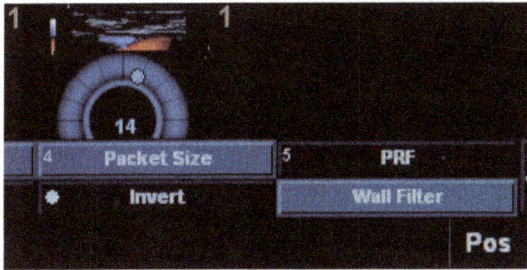

FIGURE 5-54. Color packet size control.

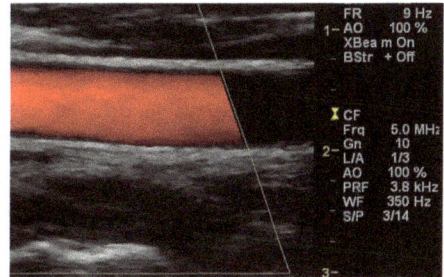

FIGURE 5-56. Color transmit frequency display. The 5.0 MHz denotes the current frequency setting of the control.

Color Line Density

The color line density settings determine the number of actual color scan lines which are acquired by the system to compose one *color frame*. Higher color scan line density improves the spatial representation of the color display, but at reduced frame rate. Lower color line density often increases the frame rate, but results in a greater amount of interpolation between lines of actual data. Color line density is set by the system depending on the transducer and preset selected. If color line density control is available (Figure 5-55), then its use can alter the color frame rate. In situations where a rapidly moving structure is of interest, the increase in fame rate may be beneficial to improve the temporal resolution of the movement. The sonographer should be aware of possible degradation of the color image if the line density is decreased by too large an amount.

Color Transmit frequency

The transmit frequency is set by default depending on the transducer and application preset selected. A control for transmit frequency may be available; in which case transmit frequency may be optimized beyond the preset value. Raising the transmitted frequency above the system default is typically not practical, as color penetration will decrease and the likelihood of color aliasing will increase. However, lowering the color transmit frequency allows greater penetration of the color pulses and may result in the ability to visualize an area of plaque within a vessel. If a user-adjustable control is available on the system, two or three settings are designated, such as "R" for resolution and "P" for penetration. A third setting, if present, is typically represented by a character either "G" for general or "N" for normal (Figure 5-56).

Color Persistence

The color persistence, or frame averaging, varies the length of time that the color information from a single frame remains on the screen. The real-time image of blood flow appears "smoother" and less mottled as persistence is increased, while the temporal resolution is degraded somewhat. Frame averaging is most appropriate in arteries or veins in which overall structural movement is less than that of the heart. Typically the sonographer sets this control based on personal preference if color persistence is user-adjustable (Figure 5-57).

COLOR FLOW IMAGE QUALITY

Color flow image quality is characterized by four factors: motion discrimination, temporal resolution, spatial resolution, and uniformity. Color is associated with movement, but it does not necessarily indicate blood

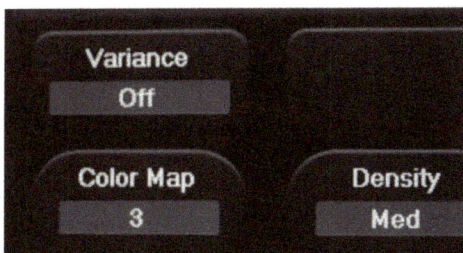

FIGURE 5-55. Color line density control set to "medium."

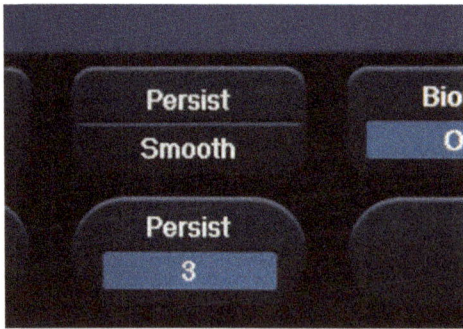

FIGURE 5-57. Color persistence control.

flow. Movement of the transducer, peristaltic motion, and cardiac motion all may contribute spurious color to the image and give an artifactual impression of flow or mask the presence of true flow. The ability to distinguish moving blood from moving tissue and at the same time depict subtle flow patterns is the ultimate goal. Low-frequency shifts from slowly moving tissue may be selectively removed with a color wall filter. Unfortunately, this technique is not completely effective in eliminating high-amplitude, low-frequency Doppler shifts associated with vessel wall movement. Also, the wall filter excludes low-velocity components, which may possibly represent slow-moving blood flow. To better differentiate flowing blood from stationary fluid and moving soft tissue, motion discrimination examines motion dynamics. Tissue and flowing blood exhibit time-varying patterns of movement, which are distinctive with respect to their source.

Temporal resolution, the ability to accurately depict movement in real time, depends on the frame rate (how often the motion is intermittently sampled). Color scan line density, width of the color field of view, packet size, and scan range affect the frame rate. High frame rate is achieved at a loss of lateral resolution (low color line density), diminished precision of the mean frequency measurements (small packet size), or limited field of view (reduced color box size).

Spatial resolution is defined by the spatial sampling by the ultrasonic field (spatial pulse length, beam width related to focusing, and scan line density). Spatial filtering is a technique to diminish random color variations throughout the image. Pixels are encoded in color only if they neighbor other pixels previously encoded in color. Small vessels with weak flow must be visualized with the spatial filter inactivated. Another type of spatial filtering (sharp or smooth processing) manipulates the presentation of the boundary between color and gray-scale pixels.

The ideal standard for uniformity is that vessels with identical properties are depicted in the same manner regardless of their respective locations within the field of view; that is, vessel delineation and color pattern should not be altered by a change in position with the field of view. This requires consistent color voxel size and color scan line density throughout the field of view.

COLOR ALIASING

Aliasing in color Doppler occurs when the velocity present exceeds the color Nyquist limit in either the positive or negative flow direction. The Nyquist limit is imposed by the color PRF, which in turn depends on depth, packet size (number of pulses required per color scan line), and how many pulses for imaging and spectral Doppler are inserted between color packets (pulse groups). High velocities from deeply located structures exhibit the greatest likelihood of color aliasing.

When very rapid flow velocities in the heart or blood vessels are present, the primary function of the color is to direct the examiner to areas to be interrogated with PW or CW spectral Doppler. Unlike spectral aliasing, which is problematic and interferes with accurate velocity measurement, color aliasing is often useful to identify areas for further study. In order to minimize color aliasing, the following techniques can be applied: turn off simultaneous modes (freeze the 2D real-time mode for example), set the velocity scale to the maximum, shift the color baseline to allow increased velocity range in that direction, decrease the packet size, and/or lower the color transmit frequency. All of these maneuvers may reduce color aliasing somewhat, although in actual practice, not much effort is expended in doing this except setting the color velocity scale (color PRF) control at the maximum for the appropriate direction of flow. Color aliasing is readily

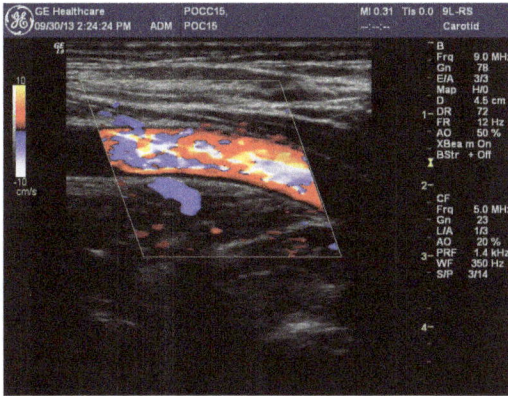

(A)

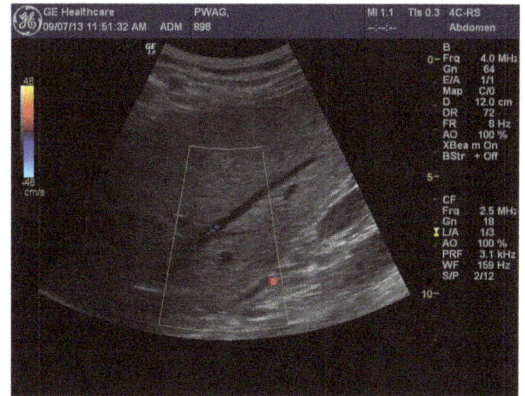

(B)

FIGURE 5-58. **(A)** Color aliasing in a normal carotid artery. Note the Nyquist limit of +/−10 cm/s mean velocity. **(B)** Color aliasing eliminated by increasing the color scale to +/−28 cm/s.

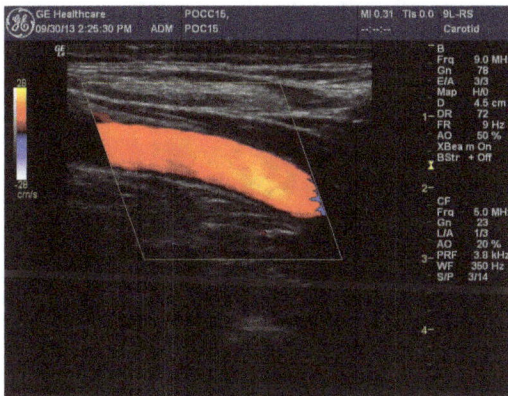

(A)

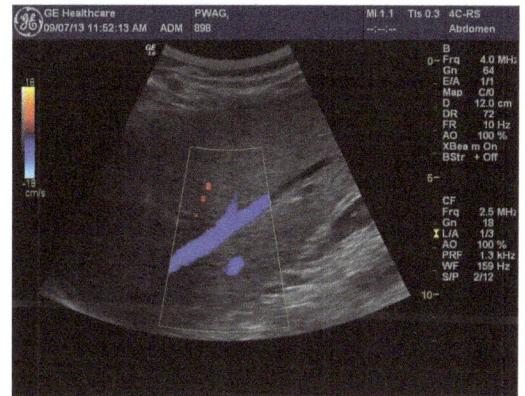

(B)

FIGURE 5-59. **(A)** Color flow image with poor hepatic venous flow visualization for color scale setting of +/−48 cm/s mean velocity. **(B)** Color flow image with good hepatic venous flow visualization for color scale setting of +/−18 cm/s mean velocity.

recognizable as a "mosaic pattern" of colors, consistent with ambiguous directional information (Figure 5-58). Color aliasing is a valuable tool for sampling placement with PW or CW spectral Doppler.

DETECTION OF SLOW FLOW

At the opposite end of the spectrum from aliasing is the ability to detect slow flow which is present in most veins and certain arteries. Using the maximum available color velocity scale often does not depict low-velocity flow. Therefore, where detection of slow flow is necessary, the velocity scale should be set to a lower value (Figure 5-59).

BENEFITS AND LIMITATIONS

The major advantage of color flow imaging is the ability to evaluate global blood flow, particularly over a large area. The detection of abnormal flow is much more rapid compared with other Doppler techniques. Identified flow abnormalities, once localized with color, may then be evaluated with PW or CW spectral Doppler for quantitative velocity information.

Diagnostic criteria unique to color Doppler have developed which cannot be easily duplicated with spectral Doppler. Color flow imaging can provide a two-dimensional representation of the direction, width, and extent of high-velocity jets such as may be seen in carotid stenosis, aortic valvular stenosis, and valvular insufficiency. A more accurate and more rapid assessment of the extent of these areas of high-velocity flow can be obtained than by spectral Doppler velocity information alone.

Color Doppler can expedite the precise placement of the spectral Doppler angle-correct marker for an off-axis stenotic jet in critical carotid stenosis. Angle correction performed in this way with the use of color may allow more precise measurement of systolic and diastolic velocities in the quantification of percent stenosis; however, the technique of angle correction with the color flow image instead of the vessel walls is not universally accepted.

Although the advantages of color flow imaging are significant, the sonographer must understand its limitations as well. Most importantly, absence of color within a vessel does not necessarily mean that no flow is present. Several important technical factors may affect whether color appears within the vessel in the presence of flow. The potential pitfalls of color flow imaging are summarized below:

- Color flow imaging is angle dependent. Color Doppler is dependent on proper angle to flow in the same manner as PW or CW spectral Doppler. The color angle to flow can be somewhat more difficult to appreciate than in spectral Doppler. Because the color box covers a wide area rather than a single line of sight as with spectral Doppler, the angle to flow may change continuously across the lateral dimension of the color box. Flow within a vessel may be shown in color at one end of the color box, while another segment of the same vessel may be depicted with no color (Figure 5-60). The sonographer can gain a better appreciation of the color angle to flow at any point within the color box by mentally drawing a series of lines across the box that are parallel with the sides of the box (Figure 5-61).

- Color velocity scale may be set improperly. Slow flow may not be visualized with high color velocity scale settings. For example, a

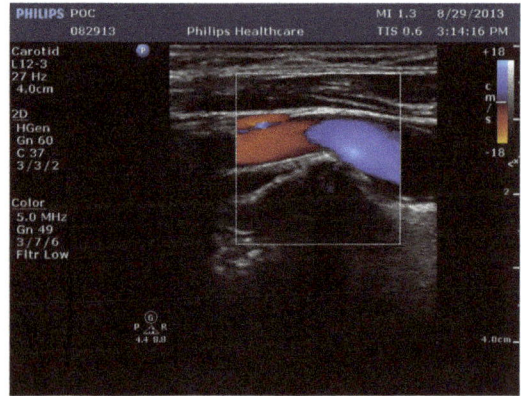

FIGURE 5-60. Unidirectional flow in a curved vessel is misrepresented in the color image by the changing angle to flow across the field of view.

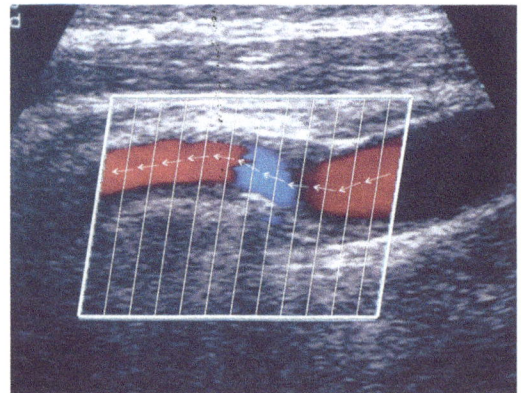

FIGURE 5-61. Color flow image of carotid bifurcation with color box and imaginary lines parallel with the sides of the box. Direction of flow is shown as parallel to the vessel wall for each line.

vertebral artery in a cerebrovascular duplex examination often requires a lower color scale setting than that used for the carotid bifurcation (Figure 5-62).

- Color gain and/or output power may be set too low. Vessels with flow are not depicted in color since the signal level does not exceed the color threshold (Figure 5-63).

- Attenuation from intervening calcific deposits may not allow penetration of the sound beam (Figure 5-64).

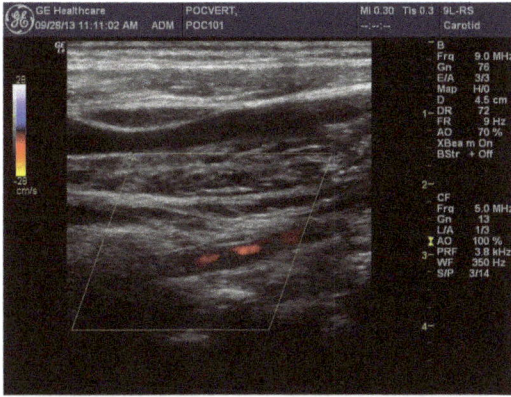

(A)

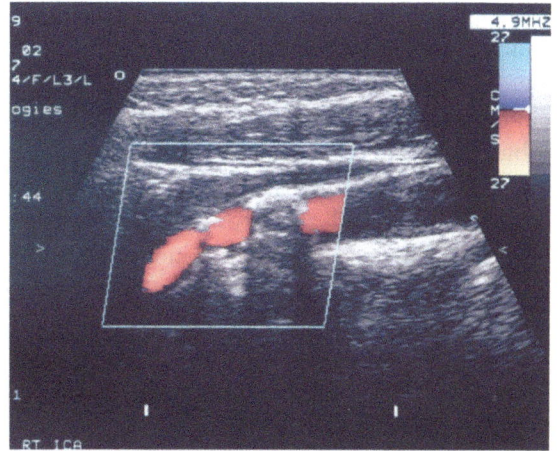

(B)

FIGURE 5-62. **(A)** Color flow image of vertebral artery with little apparent flow at color scale setting of +/−32 cm/s. **(B)** Color filling of vertebral artery with color scale setting of +/−18 cm/s.

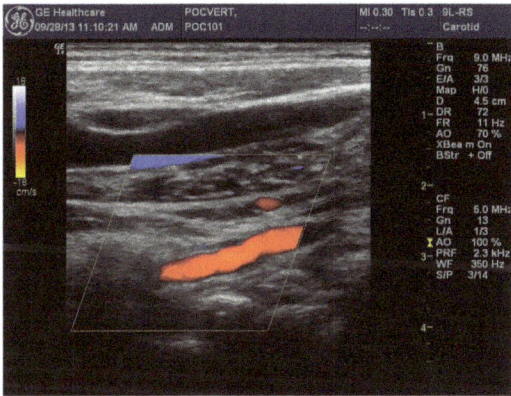

FIGURE 5-63. Color flow image of carotid artery showing no color at low color gain setting.

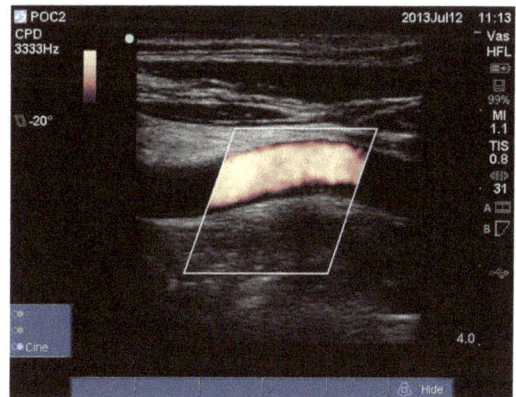

FIGURE 5-64. Color flow image of carotid plaque with shadowing. The attenuation artifact causes portions of the internal carotid artery to be displayed without color.

POWER DOPPLER IMAGING

Power Doppler imaging portrays the intensity (amplitude) of the Doppler signal without an indication of the flow velocity or direction (Figure 5-65). The Doppler signal intensity depends on the number of RBCs within the sampled volume and the attenuation by tissue along the sampling path. Power Doppler emphasizes the quantity of blood flow. The autocorrelation detector yields the total power of the Doppler signal in addition to the mean flow velocity.

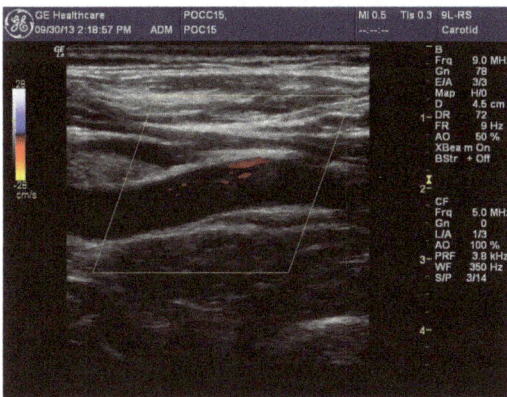

FIGURE 5-65. Power Doppler image of the common carotid artery.

Consequently, on many scanners the operator can switch easily between color flow imaging (velocity presentation) to power Doppler imaging.

Because all phase shifts (moving reflectors) contribute to the amplitude signal, power Doppler imaging is essentially nondirectional and therefore not subject to aliasing. The total power Doppler signal is relatively independent of the insonation angle except at 90 degrees. However, because the color coding does not indicate the velocity or direction of flow, pulsatility and flow reversal cannot be evaluated. Color flow imaging or spectral Doppler is required to provide velocity and directional information.

Vessel wall definition is usually improved with power Doppler imaging. Compare the relative signals arising from a sampling volume near the vessel wall with one partially overlapping the vessel wall. In color flow imaging, velocity measurements will be nearly the same, because both sampling volumes contain moving RBCs. Pixels are displayed in similar shades of color. However, for the power Doppler measurements, the total number of RBCs is very different, creating a much lower signal for the sampling volume that includes the vessel wall. Pixels are now displayed in contrasting shades of color.

The major advantage of power Doppler imaging is the ability to differentiate between regions with flow and no flow. This is usually described as increased sensitivity to depict small vessels in color, which is derived from expanded dynamic range to extend the color priority to weaker signals. Increased persistence is also employed to image flow in small vessels. Tissue motion (e.g., heart) often creates flash artifacts, which limits the applicability of this imaging mode to regions where tissue motion is more subdued, such as the liver or kidney tissue. The characteristics of power Doppler imaging are summarized in Table 5-5.

TABLE 5-5 • Characteristics of Power Doppler Imaging

Advantages	Disadvantages
Correlates with the quantity of blood flow	Subject to motion artifacts
Visualization of flow in small vessels	No velocity information
Independent of flow direction	No directional information
Independent of velocity	Low temporal resolution
Reduced Doppler angle dependence	Qualitative observations
No aliasing	
Good lumen definition	

References

Hedrick WR: Technology for diagnostic sonography, St. Louis, 2013, Elsevier.

Hedrick WR, Hykes DL: Doppler Physics and Instrumentation: A Review. Journal of Diagnostic Medical Sonography 4, 109–120, 1988.

Hedrick WR, Hykes DL: Color Doppler Imaging: Imaging Parameters and Image Quality. Journal of Diagnostic Medical Sonography 8, 180–186, 1992.

Hedrick WR, Hykes DL: Autocorrelation Detection in Color Doppler Imaging: A Review. Journal of Diagnostic Medical Sonography 11, 16–22, 1995.

Hedrick WR, Hykes DL, Starchman DE: Ultrasound physics and instrumentation, ed 4, St. Louis, 2005, Elsevier.

Kremkau FW: Diagnostic ultrasound: principles and instruments, ed 8, Philadelphia, 2011, WB Saunders.

Zagzebski JA: Essentials of ultrasound physics, St Louis, 1996, Mosby-Year Book.

6

Normal Blood Flow in Arteries and Veins

OBJECTIVES

- To understand the principles that govern blood flow in the arterial and venous systems.
- To recognize high-resistance and low-resistance flow patterns.
- To understand the significance of altered resistance patterns in arteries.

- To comprehend the factors that influence venous blood flow and characteristics of normal venous waveforms.
- To recognize venous waveforms that do not exhibit normal flow patterns.

KEY TERMS

Blunted velocity profile
Conduit vessel
Laminar flow
Parabolic velocity profile

Resistance vessel
Transmural pressure
Static filling pressure

CHARACTERISTICS OF BLOOD FLOW IN NORMAL ARTERIES

Flowing blood obeys the same principles of flow as do all fluids. Blood travels through arteries in a series of layers, a pattern known as laminar flow. The outermost layer of blood, adjacent to the vessel wall, moves very slowly due to friction with the wall itself. Subsequent layers increase in velocity, until flow in the center of the vessel is at the highest velocity (assuming the vessel is relatively straight and uniform in diameter). Laminar flow is the most energy-efficient manner in which the blood may flow through the vessel. The pattern of gradually increasing velocity from the

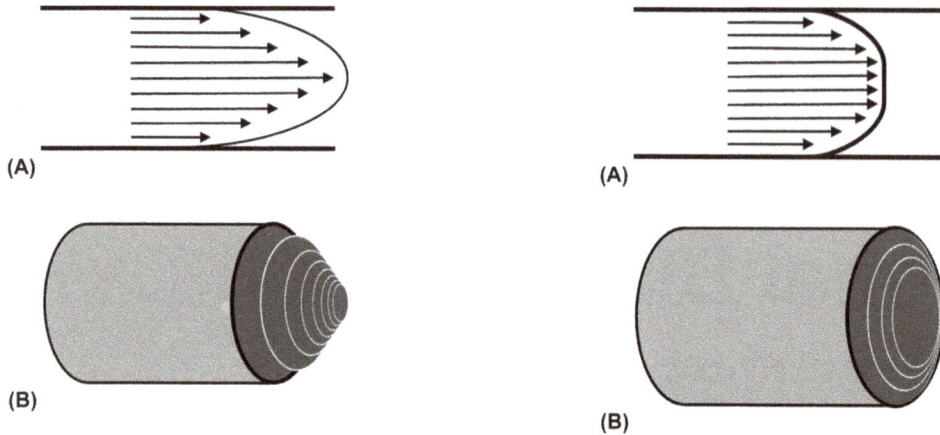

FIGURE 6-1. (**A**) Parabolic velocity profile. (**B**) 3D drawing of the parabolic velocity profile.

vessel wall to the center of the lumen is described as a parabolic velocity profile (Figures 6-1 A and B). Most arteries in the body deviate somewhat from the parabolic velocity profile due to the pulsatile nature of the flow and the relatively short length of vessels. This disparity results in a more "flattened velocity profile" or blunted velocity profile in which a large core of the central layers flows at nearly the same velocity. Thus, this flow pattern is known as "plug flow" (Figure 6-2).

Flow through a tube (in this case, a vessel) is quantified by *Poiseuille's equation* (Figure 6-3), which expresses the volume of fluid (blood) flow as proportional to the pressure differential across the tube "p_1-p_2" and the radius "r" of the tube to the fourth power, as well as inversely proportional to the viscosity "n" of the fluid and the tube length "L." For practical purposes, in the human body, blood vessels can be considered "short" tubes (in contrast to a 50-ft pipe, for example). Therefore, differences in vessel lengths have minimal effect on the volume of blood flow. The same can be said for viscosity, as the body temperature and hematocrit are relatively constant in an individual human being, and do not greatly vary from individual to individual.

From a hemodynamic consideration, vessels in the body fall into one of two categories. Conduit vessels are the larger vessels that carry the blood toward its destination and resistance vessels

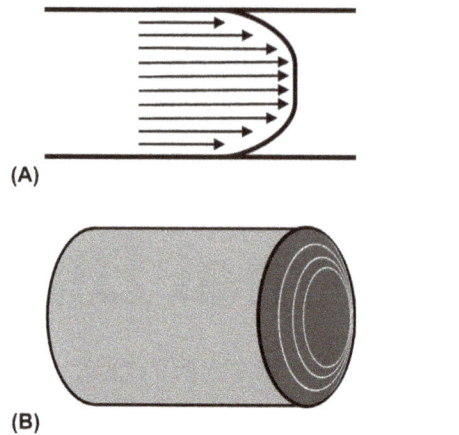

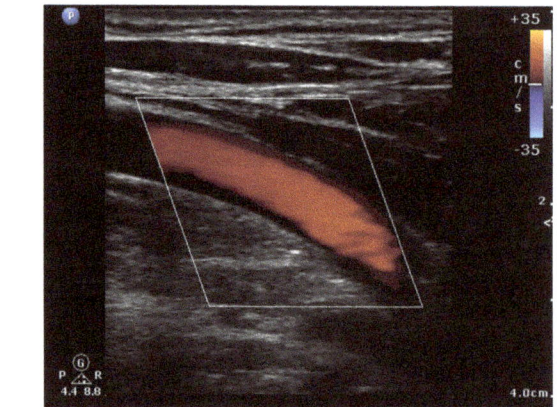

FIGURE 6-2. (**A**) Flattened velocity profile or plug flow. (**B**) 3D drawing of the plug flow. (**C**) Color flow image demonstrating the flattened velocity profile. Note the darker shades of red near the vessel walls denoting lower velocities and brighter shades toward the center of the vessel.

Poiseuille's Law

$$Q = \frac{\pi (p_1 - p_2)\, r^4}{8Ln}$$

FIGURE 6-3. Poiseuille's equation.

make up the microcirculation in tissues. Resistance vessels have the ability, through hormonal regulation of the vessel diameter, to increase and decrease resistance to flow to an organ or tissue. Thus, the flow patterns within normal conduit vessels have little to do with the vessels themselves, but instead depend on the state of the downstream resistance vessels. Flow through a normal conduit vessel, then, is determined by the pressure generated proximal to the vessel by the heart and the pressure/resistance to flow of the downstream resistance vessels. (Gravity and hydrostatic pressure also play a role).

This pressure relationship is represented in Poiseuille's equation as "p_1-p_2." Changes in either the action of the heart (p_1) or in the downstream resistance vessels (p_2) affect the flow patterns through the conduit vessel. The vessels that are examined sonographically such as carotid, femoral, hepatic, renal, and mesenteric arteries are all conduit vessels in function. When evaluating flow through one of these vessels with a Doppler instrument, knowledge of flow patterns associated with both normal and abnormal conditions is essential.

LOW-RESISTANCE WAVEFORMS

A Doppler sample obtained within a vessel such as the internal carotid or the renal artery has a waveform that indicates low downstream resistance. A low-resistance waveform exhibits forward flow in both systole and diastole (Figure 6-4).

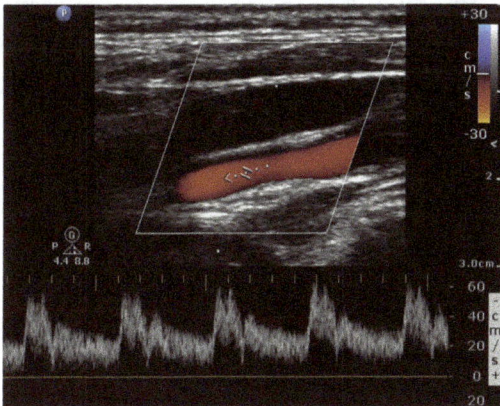

FIGURE 6-4. A low-resistance waveform with forward flow in both systole and diastole.

In a normal state, the microcirculation within most soft-tissue organs should maintain continuous low resistance to flow and therefore, the conduit arteries supplying these organs should always exhibit a low-resistance waveform. A decrease or absence of diastolic flow in the internal carotid, renal, or hepatic arteries indicates either an abnormal state in the organ such as a cerebral infarct, renal failure, or cirrhosis, or a mechanical obstruction within the vessel itself. Further Doppler evaluation of the vessel and the organ where possible should indicate which of the two possible etiologies is the correct one.

HIGH-RESISTANCE WAVEFORMS

A Doppler sample obtained within the common femoral or the subclavian artery yields a waveform that indicates high downstream resistance at rest. In a high-resistance waveform, there is little or no diastolic flow, because the downstream (p_2) pressure/resistance is actually higher than the diastolic pressure proximally (p_1). Blood is "pushed" down the artery by the pressure gradient during systole, resulting in the major component of forward flow in the waveform. As systolic pressure decreases with the onset of the diastolic phase, the forward flow drops back to zero and actually reverses briefly before reaching equilibrium through a series of small forward and reverse flow events until the flow ceases completely. These small forward and reverse events occur as a result of the elasticity, or *compliance* of the artery wall. Forward flow resumes with the next systolic phase, and the sequence is repeated. This type of high-resistance waveform is called a *triphasic* waveform, as it typically contains a forward-reverse-forward sequence (Figure 6-5).

HORMONE-MEDIATED CHANGES IN RESISTANCE

Some conduit arteries may exhibit a high-resistance waveform in the resting state but change to a low-resistance waveform as a result of some physiologic

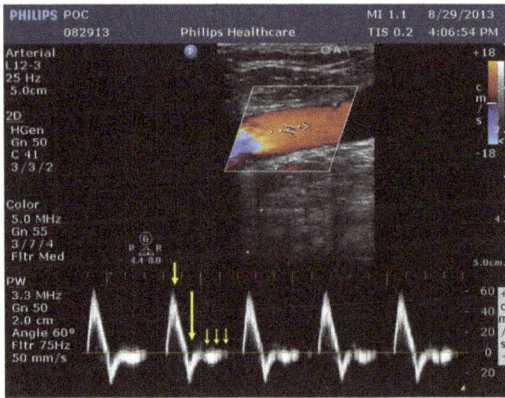

(A)

FIGURE 6-5A. The triphasic waveform. Note the large component of forward flow in systole (arrow at waveform peak), the reverse flow phase (large arrow), and the brief return to forward flow followed by several small oscillations and then zero flow in this femoral artery (small arrows). The forward flow phase was captured during this color flow image acquisition, resulting in the red color within the vessel.

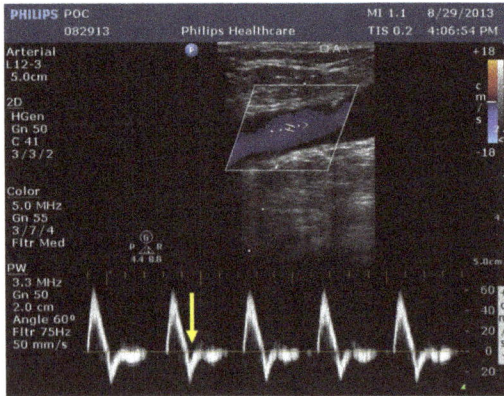

(B)

FIGURE 6-5B. The reverse flow phase (arrow on spectral waveform) was captured during this color flow image acquisition, resulting in the blue color within the vessel. In live real-time color flow imaging, the red-blue-red-blue sequence occurs very rapidly, and the reversed phase appears as only a "flash" of blue color.

change involving the tissues downstream. Most notable are the arteries that supply the skeletal muscles or the digestive tract.

Exercise of the extremity lowers the downstream (p_2) pressure/resistance in order to elicit an increase in oxygenated blood to the muscles. Therefore, Doppler

examination of blood flow in conduit arteries proximal to the skeletal muscles (such as the subclavian artery in the arm or the femoral artery in the leg) reveals evidence of decreased downstream resistance in the form of an increase in diastolic flow. After a period of rest, the (p_2) pressure/resistance again increases to the level of the resting state, and the Doppler waveform in the proximal conduit arteries returns to a characteristic high-resistance pattern (Figures 6-6). If the Doppler evaluation of the vessel shows an *absence* of this physiologic response to exercise, this is again an indicator of the presence of a disease process.

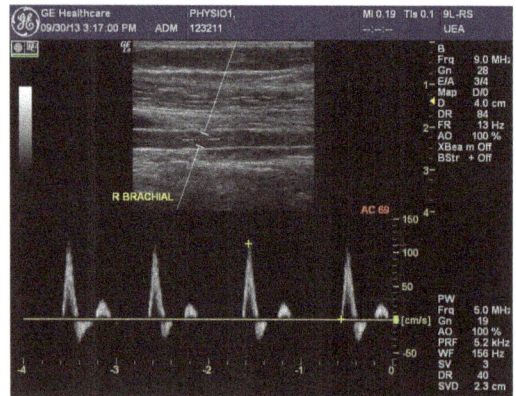

(A)

FIGURE 6-6A. Brachial artery in the resting state showing the characteristic high-resistance, triphasic waveform.

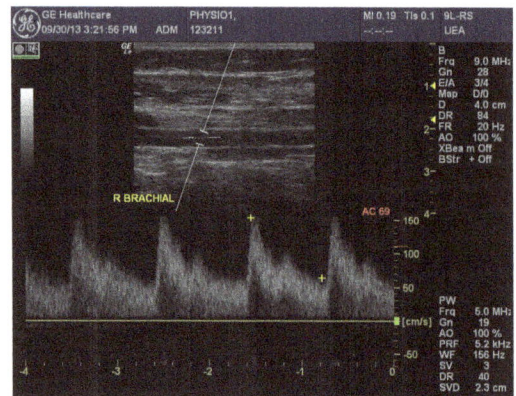

(B)

FIGURE 6-6B. Brachial artery after 5 minutes of cuff occlusion. An increase in diastolic flow occurs immediately after release of the cuff.

Mesenteric vessels exhibit a high-resistance waveform in the preprandial (fasting) state. After a meal is ingested, the (p_2) resistance decreases, thereby allowing increased blood flow to the gut for digestion. The high-resistance waveform with minimal diastolic flow within the superior mesenteric artery during fasting (resting) is shown in Figure 6-7A. In the postprandial state, the diastolic flow within the artery has dramatically increased due the physiologic response to the ingested meal (Figure 6-7B).

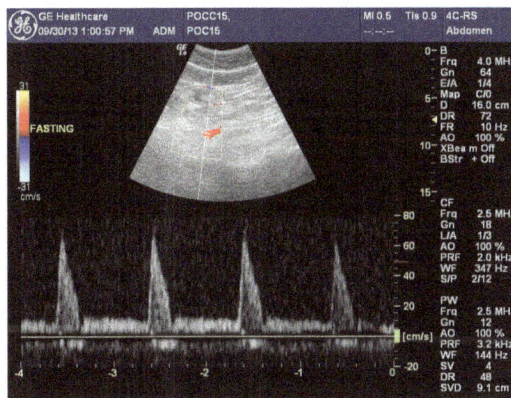

(A)

FIGURE 6-7A. Superior mesenteric artery waveform obtained in the fasting state. Note the high-resistance waveform with minimal diastolic flow.

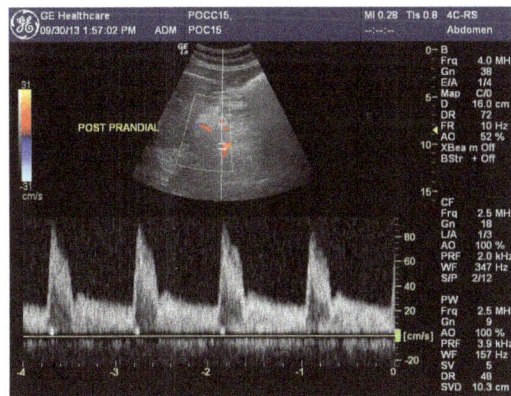

(B)

FIGURE 6-7B. After a meal the diastolic flow in superior mesenteric artery has dramatically increased due to the physiologic lowering of the p_2 pressure.

DIASTOLIC FLOW AS A PREDICTOR OF DISEASE STATES

The presence or absence of disease within a vessel or within the organ/tissues being supplied by the vessel can be confidently predicted by the sonographer with a thorough understanding of arterial hemodynamics. In an artery in which a high-resistance waveform is expected at rest, an increase in diastolic flow along with other associated changes in the waveform strongly suggests the presence of atherosclerotic disease. For the renal artery in which a low-resistance state normally exists, the presence of a high-resistance waveform strongly suggests the presence of renal artery stenosis or renal failure. These topics will be discussed in greater depth in Chapter 8.

BLOOD FLOW IN NORMAL VEINS

The primary function of the veins is the return of deoxygenated blood to the heart (or in the case of the pulmonary veins, oxygenated blood). The venous system also plays an important role in the regulation of body temperature and fluid volume, as well as acting as a storage reservoir for blood. The veins are elastic-walled, collapsible tubes, which frequently exist in the body in a partially collapsed state due to the relatively low pressure within the veins. Blood flow tends to be more a function of factors external to the veins themselves because of low intravascular pressure. Normal venous blood flow in an unobstructed vein should be phasic (varying with intrathoracic pressure during respiration) (Figure 6-8).

Forward or *antegrade* direction of flow is maintained in the veins by the function of venous valves that, when functioning properly, do not allow reversed blood flow. Valve cusps are seated within the valve sinuses in the vein walls (Figure 6-9).

Venous Pressure

Venous pressure is composed of the residual intravascular pressure created by the pumping of the

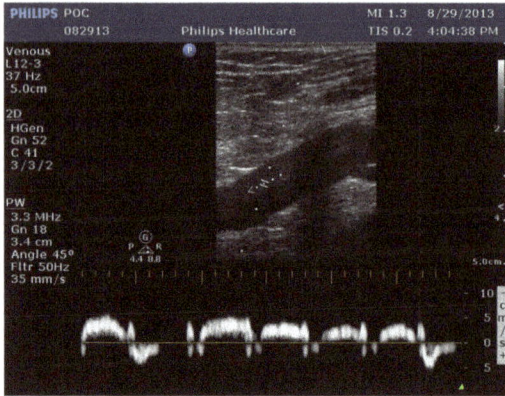

FIGURE 6-8. Fluctuating intrathoracic pressure during respiration induces phasicity in venous blood flow.

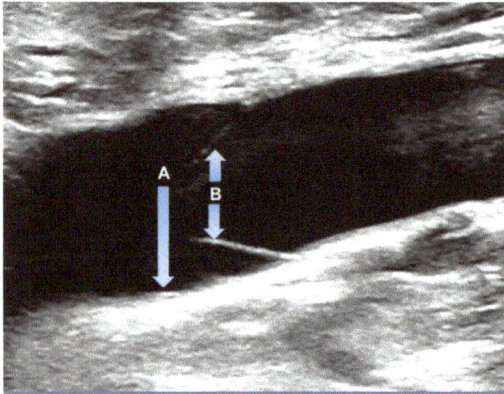

FIGURE 6-9. Venous valve cusps (**B** arrows) and venous valve sinus (**A** arrow).

left ventricle, hydrostatic pressure produced by the weight of the column of blood, and static filling pressure. *Intravascular venous pressure* attributable to the pumping action of the heart is very low, on the order of 15 mm Hg; and further shows no evidence of the pulsatile flow that is present within the arterial system. (Indeed, pulsatile veous flow is characteristic of several abnormal states such as congestive heart failure or arterio-venous fistula). Because the pressure within the vessel is low, veins are not fully distended into a cylidrical shape, but frequently exist in a partially collapsed state that varies somewhat with respiration.

Minor changes in intravascular venous pressure can cause an enormous variation in the venous volume. Figure 6-10 shows a transverse image of the common femoral vein in a partially collapsed state. Increased intrathoracic pressure created by a Valsalva maneuver causes the vein to become fully distended (Figure 6-10B).

As in the arteries, hydrostatic pressure is increased for veins below the heart and is decreased for veins above the position of the heart, a condition that occurs when the body is in an upright position. A 6 ft man standing erect has approximately +110 mm Hg hydrostatic pressure added to *both* the arterial and venous pressure at the level of the ankles. Thus, the balance between arterial and venous pressure remains constant with different patient positions.

Static filling pressure is a significant contributor to venous pressure only when increased volume distends the lumen to its full circular shape. When the vein walls are fully distended, any further increase in blood volume results in a rapid increase in venous pressure within the already-distended vein. An example of increased venous pressure due to static filling pressure would be a person with venous valvular incompetence standing in an erect position. The veins in the legs are already distended because of the hydrostatic pressure achieved in the standing

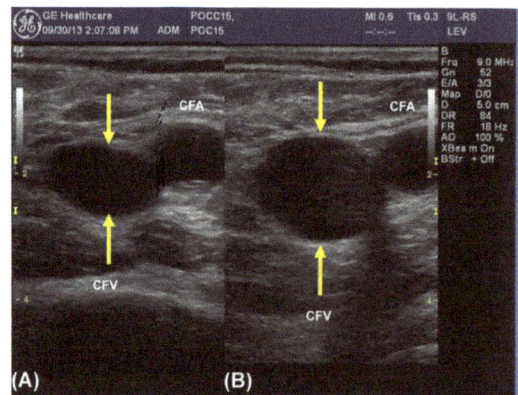

FIGURE 6-10. (**A**) Transverse image of the common femoral vein in partially collapsed state. (**B**) Fully distended vein with increased intrathoracic pressure created by a Valsalva maneuver.

position; incompetent (leaking) valves proximally cause a backflow of venous blood into the leg veins, greatly increasing the pressure.

Transmural pressure is the difference between the intralumenal pressure and the tissue pressure external to the vein. Intralumenal pressure acts to expand the vein, while external tissue pressure acts to collapse the vein. External tissue pressure may be in the form of soft tissue, muscular contraction, or mass exerting extrinsic pressure on the vein (in fact, a distended urinary bladder can exert enough pressure to reduce flow in the iliac veins), or a manual limb compression done by an examiner with hand or transducer.

Intralumenal pressure may increase or decrease with respiration, abdominal contraction (Valsalva), patient/limb position, venous valvular insufficiency, or intrinsic obstruction such as thrombus. Higher intrathoracic pressure can be seen with a Valsalva maneuver resulting in a brief decrease or stoppage of venous return. A Valsalva maneuver performed in this way may reverse the blood flow in veins in which a valve or valves are not functioning adequately. Thus, the Valsalva maneuver is used diagnostically to evaluate for the presence of venous valvular insufficiency (Figure 6-11).

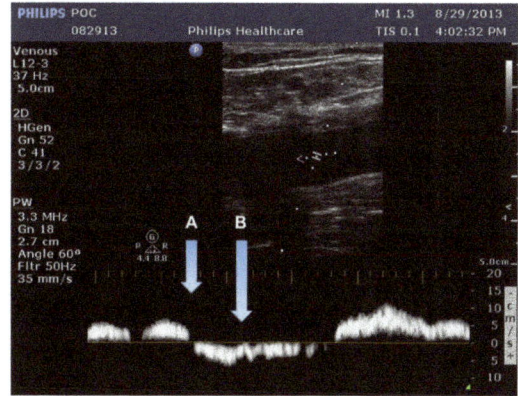

FIGURE 6-11. Flow reversal in the common femoral vein in response to Valsalva maneuver. Initiation of the Valsalva (arrow A). Flow reversal through the nonfunctioning valve(s) (arrow B).

References

Hedrick WR: Technology for diagnostic sonography, St. Louis, 2013, Elsevier.

Hedrick WR, Hykes DL, Starchman DE: Ultrasound physics and instrumentation, ed 4, St. Louis, 2005, Elsevier.

Nichols W, O'Rourke M: McDonalds's blood flow in arteries: theoretical experimental, and clinical principles, ed 5, New York, 2005, Oxford University Press, Inc.

Pellerito J, Polak J: Introduction to vascular sonography, ed 6, Philadelphia, 2012, Elsevier.

7

Types of Devices

OBJECTIVES

- To understand the different capabilities of hand-held versus portable console scanners.

- To recognize the equipment requirements for various sonographic applications.

KEY TERMS

Hand-held scanner
Portable console scanner

Scanning window
Transducer Footprint

INTRODUCTION

Requirements for portable ultrasound equipment are based primarily on the proposed applications. The cost of point-of-care scanners ranges from around $6000 for a portable "hand-held" scanner to well over $100,000 for a full-featured laptop system. The purchaser must match the capabilities (and price) of the point-of-care system with the expected clinical use. If the objective is to provide a high-end, full-range diagnostic service capable of cardiac, obstetrics, abdominal, breast, and musculoskeletal (MSK) imaging, a low-cost scanner will not be adequate.

TRANSDUCER APPLICATIONS

In Chapter 3, six types of transducers have been discussed. Each transducer type is intended for specific applications and has unique features and image formats. The scanner must accommodate not only the transducer itself, but also the electronics to support that transducer. For example, a phased sector transducer requires different hardware and electronics than a linear array transducer. Essentially, the design of an ultrasound unit is based on the intended transducers of use. Transducers can be grouped more generally into two main categories: (1) sector type and (2) linear array.

Sector-Type Transducers

The sector (or phased array) transducer generates a cone-shaped image format with the sound source originating from a small apex. The area of the transducer face that contacts the patient is called the transducer footprint. A small transducer footprint is advantageous for applications for which there is very limited access at the skin surface. The most common use of sector transducers is imaging of the heart. Sound enters the body via a small scanning window and the two-dimensional field of view widens with scan depth. Indeed, most cardiac scanning would not be possible without sector technology. The phased array is also utilized for intercostal scanning within the abdomen.

Sector transducers are required for adult and pediatric cardiac scanning, but also can perform abdominal, gynecological, and basic obstetrical scanning reasonably well. Sectors are not suitable for musculoskeletal, breast, or thyroid (small parts) imaging because field of view is narrowed in the near field and maximum frequency is generally limited to 5 MHz. They are also inadequate for most vascular applications. Cardiac applications ideally require two transducers with different frequency ranges for both adult and pediatric use. The majority of hand-held units utilize sector technology (Figure 7-1).

Linear Array Transducers

Linear array transducer technology encompasses multiple transducer types including the straight (flat) linear array, convex or curvilinear array, steered linear array, and vector array. These transducer types rely primarily on the same basic method for image formation, that is, the elements are excited in successive groups across the face of the transducer to create the two-dimensional image. The curvilinear array, with its curved geometry, produces a wider field of view than does a standard linear array. The vector array extends the width of the field of view by implementing phased beam steering (similar to a phased array) at the periphery. The steered linear array is capable of steering (angling) the entire image area to the left or right when necessary.

The linear array is the transducer of choice for obstetrics, gynecology, breast, superficial structures including MSK, and vascular applications (if duplex spectral Doppler is available). Abdominal scanning with a curvilinear array is now the standard of practice and this transducer can also achieve intercostal scanning of the abdomen (Figures 7-2 and 7-3). At least three separate broadband linear array transducers are necessary to perform the full complement of clinical applications: a low-frequency curvilinear array in the range of 3–5 MHz (abdomen and OB-gyn), a 7- to 10- MHz transducer with Doppler

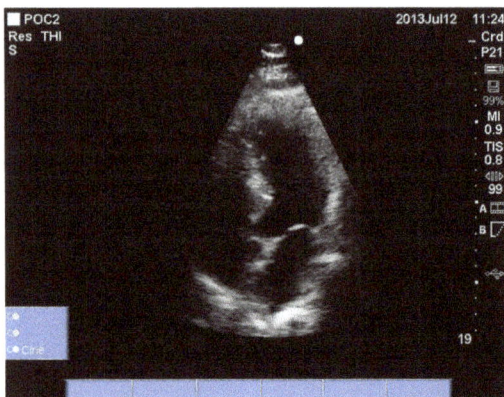

FIGURE 7-1. Sector image of heart, four-chamber view, obtained with a hand-held scanner.

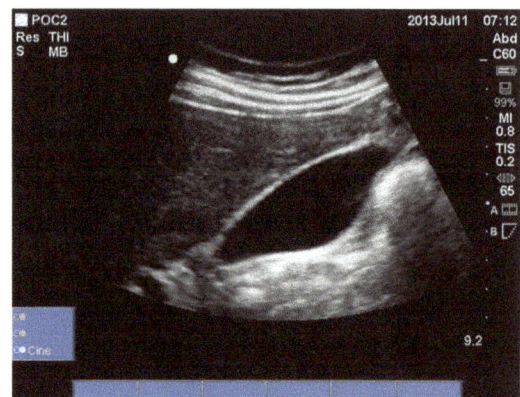

FIGURE 7-2. B-mode image of the gallbladder acquired with a curvilinear array.

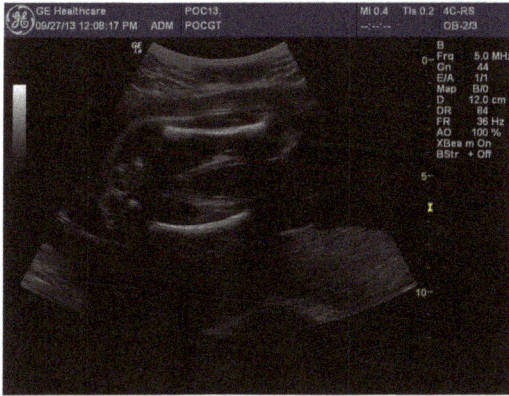

FIGURE 7-3. B-mode image of a fetus showing both femurs acquired with a curvilinear array.

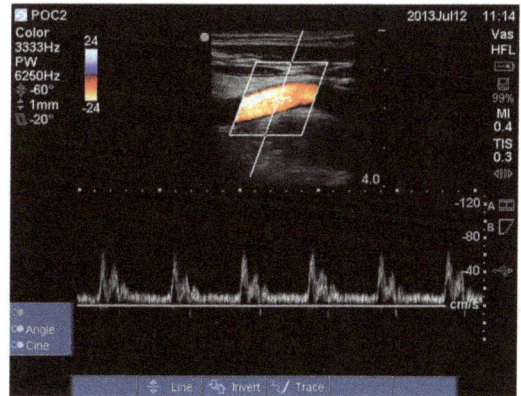

FIGURE 7-5. Color flow imaging with pulsed-wave spectral Doppler of the common carotid artery.

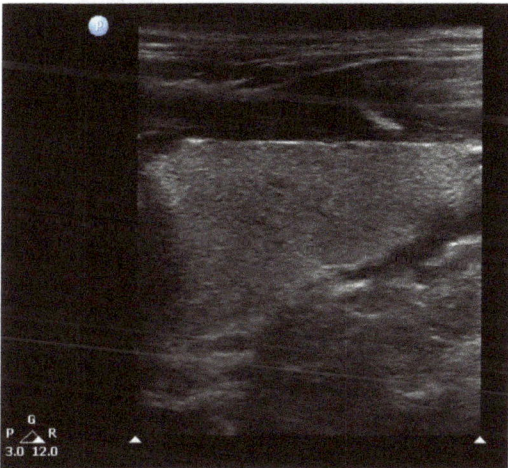

FIGURE 7-4. B-mode image of the thyroid gland acquired with linear array.

capability (vascular), and a high-frequency linear array in the 12–15 MHz range (breast, thyroid and MSK) (Figure 7-4). In addition, a dedicated OB-gyn scanner requires an endovaginal transducer as well as three-dimensional (3D) technology for obstetrical imaging. Linear array transducers are not suitable for cardiac imaging due to their large transducer footprint.

EVALUATION OF BLOOD FLOW

Most portable scanners, including hand-held models, include color flow imaging. This capability can be extremely valuable in emergency situations and in remote areas where these scanners are the only systems available.

Complete, quantitative evaluation of blood flow is achieved with spectral Doppler in pulsed-wave format. Continuous-wave format is also required if cardiac applications are included in the clinical setting. The potential purchaser must be aware that vascular applications require spectral Doppler capability, which may not be available on low-priced systems (Figure 7-5).

CONSOLE DESIGN

Point-of-care scanners on the market today can be grouped into two basic categories. Hand-held scanners are small, lightweight, and inexpensive. They are often described as the "new stethoscope" and offer basic imaging capability in a variety of situations. At the bedside, the physician or other healthcare practitioner, with proper training, can make a basic assessment of patient condition. Hand-held scanners are ideal for limited assessments, such as the FAST (focused assessment with sonography for trauma) protocol, which can be performed in an emergency environment by individuals with appropriate training. In underdeveloped countries, the most basic ultrasound imaging capability offered by hand-held scanners can make a significant contribution to patient care (Figures 7-6 and 7-7).

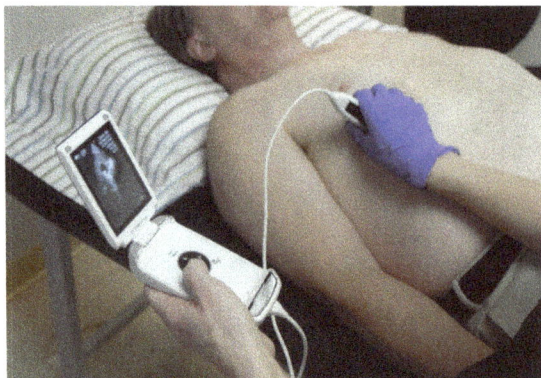

FIGURE 7-6. Scanning performed with hand-held scanner.

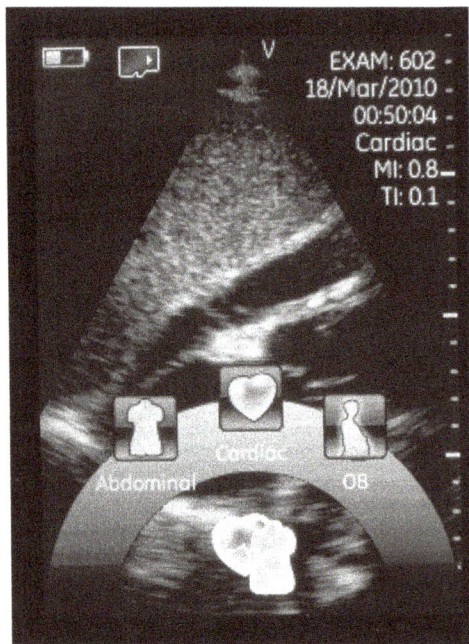

FIGURE 7-7. Application preset selector for a hand-held scanner.

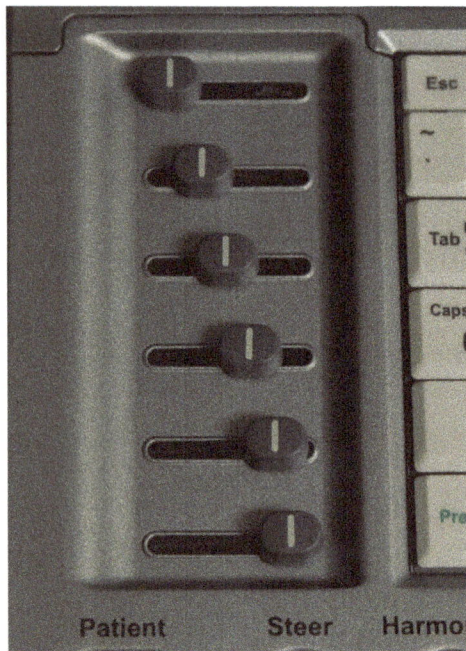

FIGURE 7-8. TGC controls in traditional slider-type configuration present on a portable console scanner.

Portable console scanners, commonly manufactured with a folding laptop design, are more robust than hand-held scanners and are intended for wide-ranging applications in the point-of-care environment. Many function as portable systems in hospitals when bedside access is required. Manufacturers of portable console scanners have adopted two different approaches in design. Some manufacturers have successfully recreated a full-sized scanner in a portable package. Most, if not all, of the controls that a sonographer would expect to find on a full-sized scanner are also available on the portable system, including TGC (time gain compensation), output power, gain, transmit frequency, variable focusing, and harmonics (Figure 7-8). Other manufacturers, notably Sonosite, have created a scanner for which many parameters including focus, transmit frequency, and output power are controlled indirectly by the operator according to transducer and examination preset

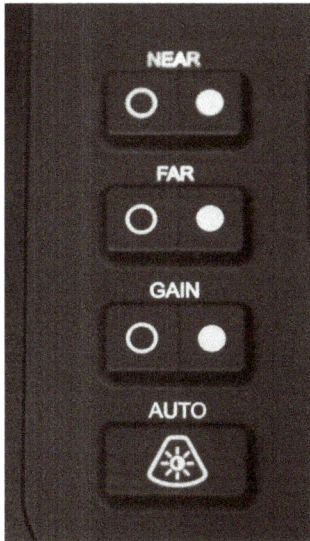

FIGURE 7-9. TGC controls utilizing push-button selectors for near gain and far gain on a portable console scanner.

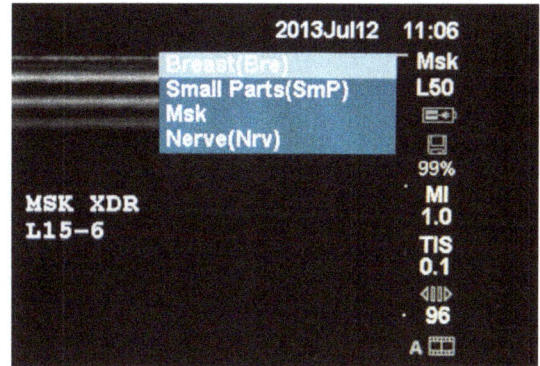

FIGURE 7-10. Application preset selection based on connected transducer for a portable console scanner.

selected (Figures 7-9 and 7-10). Both system designs work well in the point-of-care environment and the choice of scanner when purchasing should be based on intended application, image quality, ease of use, service support, and price.

References

Hedrick WR: Technology for diagnostic sonography, St. Louis, 2013, Elsevier.

Hedrick WR, Hykes DL, Starchman DE: Ultrasound physics and instrumentation, ed 4, St. Louis, 2005, Elsevier.

Kremkau FW: Diagnostic ultrasound: principles and instruments, ed 8, Philadelphia, 2011, WB Saunders.

Zagzebski JA: Essentials of ultrasound physics, St. Louis, 1996, Mosby-Year Book.

8

Doppler Evaluation of Blood Flow

OBJECTIVES

- To recognize abnormal patterns in spectral Doppler waveforms associated with various disease states.

- To learn potential techniques for the elimination of aliasing.

KEY TERMS

Flow disturbance
Laminar flow
Point of maximum stenosis

Reynolds' number
Spectral broadening
Turbulence

ARTERIAL FLOW PATTERNS

Blood flow through normal conduit arteries is *laminar* in nature, meaning that it flows in layers. As discussed in earlier chapters, laminar flow occurs because this arrangement is the most energy-efficient way for blood to move through a vessel. In laminar flow, the layers with the slowest velocities are present near the vessel walls and the fastest velocities reside in the center of the vessel lumen. As atherosclerotic disease progresses, plaque buildup

restricts the vessel lumen. Plaque buildup forms a mechanical obstruction within the artery and alters blood flow patterns within the vessel. Initially, the developing plaque creates areas of eddying (helical flow) and pooling of blood, causing mild flow disturbance. Flow disturbance, or disturbed flow, is generally accepted to mean a shift away from purely laminar flow, but without the energy losses associated with turbulence. Disturbed flow usually reverts readily back to purely laminar flow after the area causing the disturbance is passed. As long as overall

Hemodynamics of Mild Plaque
(Non-hemodynamically Significant Disease)

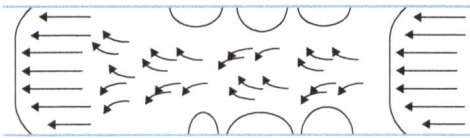

FIGURE 8-1. Blood flow through an artery with mild atherosclerotic disease shows the presence of eddy currents and a greater range of velocities, all associated with mild flow disturbance.

laminar flow is maintained, there is minimal energy loss and pressure is maintained throughout the vessel as well as downstream (Figure 8-1).

MILD FLOW DISTURBANCE

Both spectral Doppler and color flow imaging depict mild flow disturbance as an increased range of velocities present within the sampled volume. In spectral Doppler, this is manifested by a "filling in" of the *spectral window*, often described as spectral broadening (Figure 8-2). However, the peak velocities throughout the vessel remain within the normal range because plaque buildup is not sufficient to create a significant reduction of flow volume through the conduit vessel.

The measured velocities associated with a "normal velocity range" depend upon the artery. Several well-accepted tables exist for the grading of stenosis of the internal carotid artery, for example, which can be used to compare peak systolic and end-diastolic velocities obtained by spectral Doppler. Elsewhere in the body, upstream and downstream velocities are compared with the velocity in the area being interrogated to determine whether the velocity is normal or abnormal.

Disease with no elevated velocity flow is usually categorized as "mild" or "non-hemodynamically significant." Color flow imaging depicts non-hemodynamically significant disease with inverted color along the vessel walls and sometimes in the center of the vessel, depending on the locations of plaque formation (Figure 8-3). Inverted color depicts small areas of retrograde flow from eddy currents.

Flow disturbance and the resultant spectral broadening are frequently present in normal arteries in certain circumstances, such as within a curved vessel, at or near a bifurcation, and where the arterial diameter changes (e.g., carotid bulb). Therefore, spectral broadening is nonspecific for the identification of disease or the estimation of its severity (Figure 8-4).

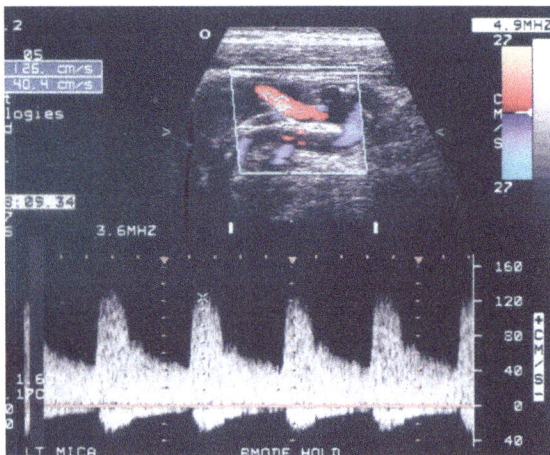

FIGURE 8-2. Filling in of the spectral window, often described as spectral broadening is demonstrated in this internal carotid artery with non-hemodynamically significant atherosclerotic disease. Note the small amount of reverse flow seen below the baseline.

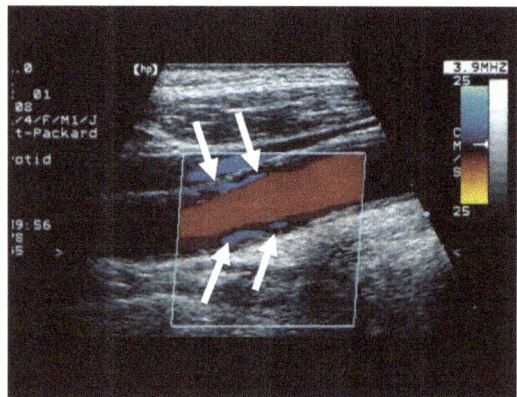

FIGURE 8-3. Color flow imaging depicts flow disturbance in non-hemodynamically significant disease as areas of inverted color (blue) along the vessel walls, and sometimes in the center of the vessel, depending on the locations of plaque formation (arrows).

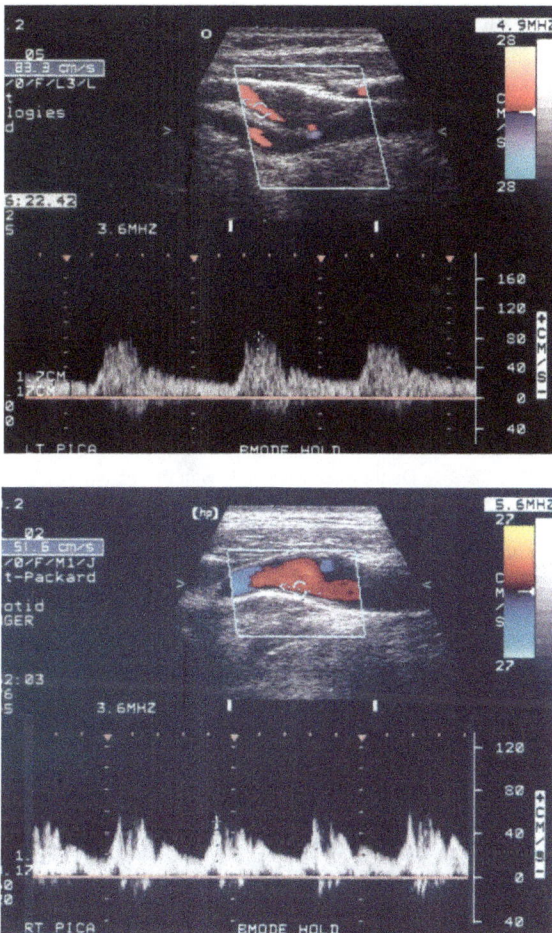

FIGURE 8-4. Two examples of flow disturbance within the normal carotid bulb. The eddy currents are indicated by areas of blue in the color flow image. Spectral broadening is present in each case. Note that the samples are taken off-center in the vessel in order to capture the highest velocity. In practice, the sample is moved back and forth across the vessel lumen until the highest forward velocity is identified.

FLOW-LIMITING ARTERIAL STENOSIS

As the plaque enlarges, the remaining luminal area decreases. To compensate for the smaller effective lumen diameter, blood velocity must increase through the narrowed region in order to maintain the same flow volume through the vessel. Blood velocities become greater as the obstruction becomes more

severe. Normal arterial velocities are typically in the range of 30–125 cm/s. In severe stenosis, velocities may exceed 500 cm/s. As high-velocity flow exits, the stenotic region, turbulence, occurs. Turbulence is characterized by the complete loss of laminar flow and movement of blood cells which is often at right angles or even 180 degrees to the axis of the vessel. Turbulent flow is sometimes described as *chaotic* flow.

The elimination of ordered laminar flow results in higher energy losses from friction, causing decreased pressure downstream from the point of stenosis. The initiation of turbulence in response to increasing velocity varies from patient to patient and from lesion to lesion. Factors that contribute to turbulence formation include viscosity of the blood, vessel diameter, velocity and direction of the stenotic jet, length of the stenotic region, and roughness of the surface of the plaque. These factors are combined in a dimensionless metric called Reynolds' number, which predicts the onset of turbulence in arterial stenosis. A Reynolds' number of around 2000 is generally considered necessary to cause turbulence; however, this is not universally true. Under certain conditions, turbulence may occur at Reynolds' numbers less than 2000 and conversely, laminar flow can be maintained at higher values.

Doppler interrogation of the diseased artery can yield several different characteristic waveforms, depending on the spatial relationship between the sampled location and the stenotic region. If the point of maximum stenosis can be identified and sampled, abnormally high velocities are apparent (Figure 8-5). Immediately distal or downstream from the stenosis, turbulent flow is punctuated by the presence of a high-velocity jet extending some distance downstream from the stenosis (Figure 8-6). The high-velocity jet may extend along an axis parallel to the vessels walls, but is often generated along a completely different direction. Color flow imaging may help delineate the true spatial composition of the high-velocity jet.

The turbulent flow may extend for a considerable distance downstream. For example, stenosis of the renal artery at its origin may result in turbulence which extends the entire length of the renal artery. When the stenosis becomes severely flow-limiting,

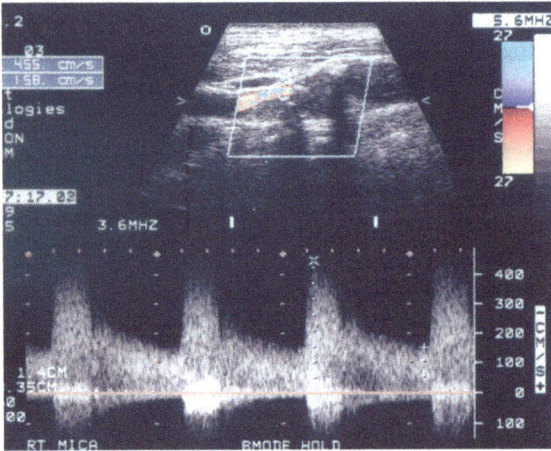

FIGURE 8-5. Doppler sample at the point of maximum stenosis showing peak systolic velocity of over 400 cm/s.

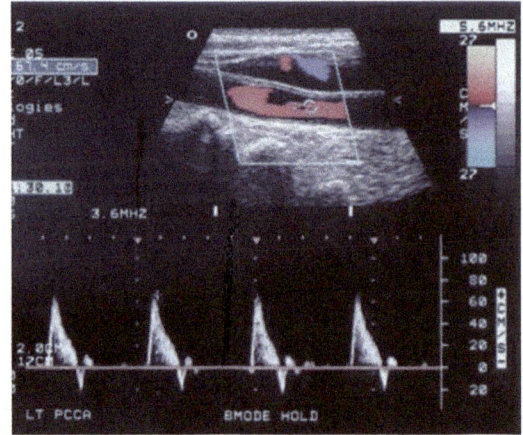

FIGURE 8-7. Decreased diastolic flow in this common carotid artery is seen proximal to (upstream from) the point of maximal stenosis. This is a result of increased resistance in the vessel caused by the downstream stenosis present in the internal carotid artery.

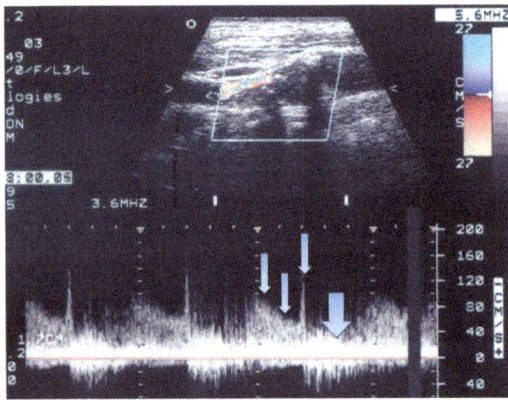

FIGURE 8-6. Doppler sample obtained immediately distal, or downstream from the stenosis, demonstrating an area of turbulent flow (large arrow) and a portion of the high-velocity jet (small arrows) extending from the stenosis for some distance downstream within the vessel.

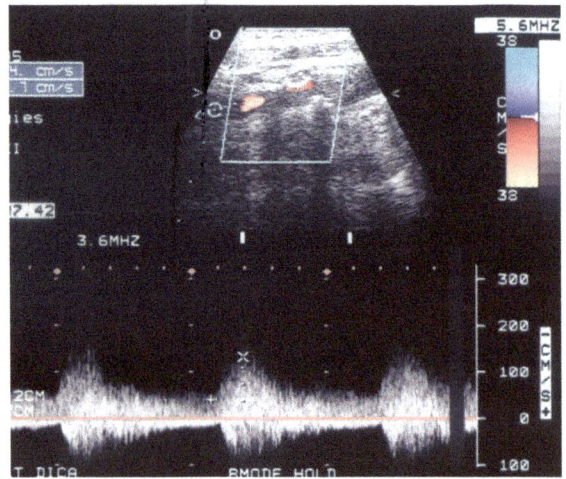

FIGURE 8-8. Doppler sample taken further downstream from the stenosis shows a delayed systolic upstroke and a delayed systolic deceleration phase. Turbulence is still evident in the Doppler spectral waveform far downstream from the stenosis.

resistance to flow is increased at the point of obstruction. This becomes apparent in the form of decreased diastolic flow in Doppler samples acquired proximally or *upstream* from the stenosis (Figure 8-7).

Doppler samples taken further downstream from the turbulent region, if obtainable, show a return to laminar flow, but with delayed systolic upstroke and delayed systolic deceleration phase (Figure 8-8). This type of flow pattern is sometimes referred to a *tardus*

parvus waveform, which, loosely translated, means "slow to rise, slow to fall."

Figure 8-9 is a diagrammatic representation of the progression of Doppler waveforms in association with severe arterial stenosis.

Hemodynamics of a Stenosis

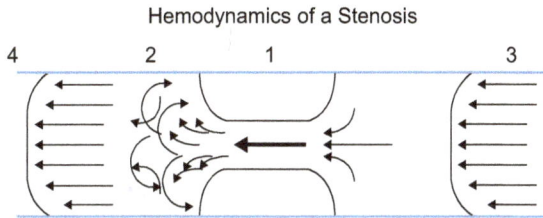

Zone 1 - Abrupt increase in velocity at PMS
Zone 2 - Abrupt decrease in velocity with turbulence
Zone 3 - Evidence of increased downstream resistance
Zone 4 - Permanent energy losses (pressure), delayed
systolic upstroke ("tardus parvus" waveform)

FIGURE 8-9. Diagrammatic representation of hemodynamically significant stenosis. Zone 1 is the point of maximal stenosis; Zone 2 represents post-stenotic turbulence at the exit of the stenosis with possible inclusion of a portion of the stenotic jet; Zone 3 represents an increase in resistance seen proximal to the stenosis; Zone 4 represents downstream return to laminar flow with tardus parvus waveform and continued evidence of flow disturbance.

ALIASING

Elevated velocities associated with high-grade arterial stenosis or with aortic or mitral valvular stenosis are particularly susceptible to aliasing (Figure 8-10). As discussed previously, the Doppler pulse repetition frequency must be at least twice the Doppler shift frequency in order to accurately record flow velocity. As flow velocities approach and then exceed the Nyquist limit, Doppler shift frequencies are no longer accurately portrayed. When this occurs, the peak systolic velocity can no longer be determined accurately. This is a serious problem because estimation of percent stenosis in vascular disease and aortic valve area in aortic valvular stenosis are heavily dependent upon the measured peak systolic velocity.

Aliasing and various approaches to remedy this problem can perhaps be better understood by classifying parameters that affect aliasing into two groups. The first group of factors are those that affect the Doppler shift frequency. The second group of factors affect the Doppler pulse repetition frequency (PRF) of the instrument. Factors that contribute to aliasing are summarized in the two groups below. Several of these factors are under the control of the sonographer.

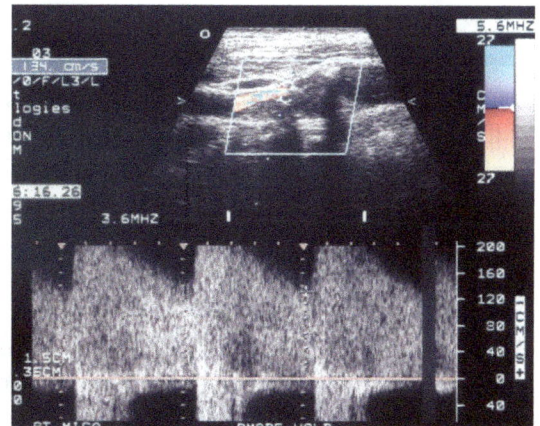

(A)

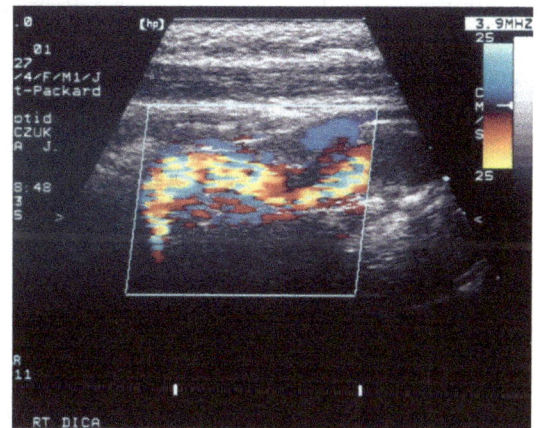

(B)

FIGURE 8-10. Examples of aliasing. (**A**) Spectral aliasing demonstrated in this PW Doppler sample of an arterial stenosis. (**B**) Color aliasing shows a characteristic "mosaic" pattern indicative of ambiguous velocity information.

Factors that affect Doppler shift frequency:

- Velocity of blood flow
- Transmitted frequency (transducer in Doppler mode)
- Doppler angle to flow (0–60 degrees)

Factors that affect the Doppler PRF:

- Velocity scale setting
- Baseline setting
- Depth of the sample volume (gate)
- "Simultaneous" modes

Velocity of Blood Flow

Velocity of the blood flow is obviously not under the control of the sonographer. Indeed, determination of flow velocity is the reason the examination is performed. However, transmit frequency and Doppler angle to flow may be altered by the sonographer, to enable the accurate measurement of flow velocity.

Transmit Frequency

Decreasing the Doppler transmit frequency correspondingly reduces the Doppler shift frequency, which becomes a potential tactic to eliminate aliasing. The Doppler transmit frequency is set by the examination preset and the selected transducer according to the transmit frequency range available in Doppler mode. Of note is that the nominal frequency of a particular probe refers only to the two-dimensional imaging frequency. For example, a transducer labeled as 6–10 MHz describes the range of real-time B-mode imaging frequencies, usually without reference to the transmit frequency utilized in the spectral Doppler or color Doppler modes.

Many point-of-care ultrasound instruments allow the operator to adjust the Doppler transmit frequency. The control for Doppler transmit frequency may be labeled "transmitted frequency" or simply as "f" and is displayed within the partition of Doppler settings when the unit is in the Doppler mode. The actual transmit frequency may be indicated, for example "2.5 MHz," or the transmit frequency settings may be indicated with nomenclature such as "low–medium–high." Another possible scheme labels the Doppler transmit frequency as "penetration–resolution" or "penetration–general–resolution," if two or three options are available. Lowering the Doppler transmit frequency causes a corresponding decrease in the Doppler shift frequency, which may reduce aliasing or eliminate it altogether. As a bonus, the lower transmit frequency may better penetrate calcified plaque within a vessel or heart valve.

Doppler Angle to Flow

A Doppler angle close to zero degrees yields the highest Doppler shift frequency from the sampled volume. (In the Doppler equation, cosine of zero degrees results in the highest absolute value for cosine of the angle, which is 1.) In some clinical applications, the sonographer has flexibility to vary the Doppler angle. For example, an arterial stenosis can often be approached from several different angles. Insonation of the vessel at a 60-degree angle has less likelihood for aliasing than does a 20-degree angle. In other situations, the sonographer has severe limitations in the manipulation of the Doppler angle, which make altering the angle to flow impractical or impossible.

Spectral Velocity Scale

Increasing and decreasing the spectral velocity scale simultaneously increases or decreases the Doppler PRF. In fact, some manufacturers label this control "Doppler PRF" or simply "PRF" (in Doppler mode). Higher Doppler pulse repetition frequency raises the Nyquist limit, possibly to a level that is sufficient to measure reflector velocity accurately. If the maximum pulse repetition frequency (the upper limit of the velocity scale control) does not remove the aliasing artifact, then one of the strategies below may work.

Spectral Baseline

Aliasing may sometimes be eliminated by lowering (or raising, depending on the flow direction) the spectral baseline, which partitions more (or all) of the available velocity scale to flow in that specific direction. This tactic presumes that there is no flow in the opposite direction (or not of interest), since it is not displayed. Changing the baseline may work alone or in combination with one of the above techniques

Depth of the Sample Volume

The PW Doppler sampling depth is determined by the distance between the transducer and the location of the sample volume (gate). As the sampling depth is increased, the necessary delay time between each transmitted pulse becomes longer and therefore, the maximum number of Doppler pulses that can be transmitted in one second (the Doppler PRF) decreases. This reduction in Doppler PRF has a direct result of lowering the Nyquist limit (Nyquist limit equals one-half the PRF).

In some circumstances, the patient position or scanning approach can be manipulated to permit a shallower sampling depth. For example, an image of the renal arteries obtained with the patient in the supine position may have a sampling depth of 16–18 cm. Repositioning the patient into a decubitus position may result in an approach in which the transducer is closer to the kidney. In this situation, the shallower sample depth enables a higher Doppler PRF, thereby increasing the Nyquist Limit.

Simultaneous Modes

Simultaneous modes, such as real-time B-mode imaging, color flow imaging, and spectral Doppler, can greatly reduce the Doppler PRF. Simultaneous modes are not actually simultaneous, but operate instead by interleaving two-dimensional imaging (color and/or B-Mode) pulses between the Doppler pulses. This theoretically reduces the Doppler PRF and can dramatically lower the Nyquist limit, depending on the instrument. The recommended practice for most situations is to freeze the B-mode and color flow image during live Doppler acquisition, which preserves the quality of the two-dimensional image and, at the same time, ensures the maximum Doppler PRF.

Combination of Techniques

In actual practice, a sonographer often utilizes a combination of the above techniques to eliminate aliasing. For example, a moderate amount of aliasing may be corrected by (1) lowering the transmit frequency, (2) raising the velocity scale to the maximum setting, and (3) moving the baseline to the top or bottom of the spectral display. In situations where increasing the Doppler angle to 60 degrees is possible and appropriate, that technique may also be part of the potential solution. Repositioning of the transducer or patient may also be employed.

CW Doppler

In the heart, aortic valvular stenosis can generate velocities above 6 m/s and must be insonated at

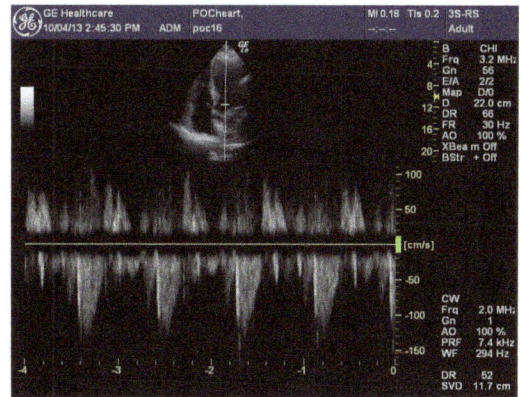

FIGURE 8-11. Continuous wave Doppler in duplex mode demonstrating flow through mitral valve and left ventricular outflow tract. CW Doppler records all velocity flow information along the sound beam path.

an angle as close as possible to 0 degrees. In such circumstances, the combination of very high velocity, the Doppler sound beam being parallel to flow (0 degrees), and deep depth of the aortic valve creates the worst possible scenario for aliasing. Eliminating PW Doppler aliasing in these situations is practically impossible. However, one solution is to localize the high-velocity valvular jet with the aid of color flow imaging and PW Doppler, and then switch to continuous-wave (CW) Doppler while in the duplex mode. Because CW Doppler has no limitation in the measurement of high Doppler shift frequencies, the accurate peak systolic velocity can often be obtained (Figure 8-11). Aortic valvular stenosis can also be evaluated with a CW Doppler non-imaging probe (pitoff probe) by sonographers experienced in this technique.

High-PRF Mode

Most ulrasound systems offer what has been termed "high-PRF" mode. High-PRF mode is a pulsed-wave (PW) mode that operates above the transmission rate for normal echo ranging and thus permits a higher Nyquist limit at a cost of some ambiguity in range resolution. However, in practical application, the compromised range resolution does not normally affect the ability to accurately display the higher velocities associated with the pathology under investigation. In high-PRF mode, the Doppler PRF is increased above the value that would normally be permitted by the given depth of the sample. In other words, subsequent Doppler pulses are transmitted without sufficient time for all of the returning echoes to have reached the tranducer. In this way, the Doppler PRF can be increased to several times the traditional value, permtting accurate display of considerably higher velocities without aliasing. Instead of just one sample volume along the beam path, there are multiple sample volumes. Doppler information is obtained from all sample volumes which is then added together to produce the resultant Doppler waveform (Figure 8-12). High-PRF mode, if available, may be activated in one of several ways, depending on the design of the system. On some scanners, high-PRF mode will have a separate on/off control that may be accessed through a soft key or menu selection. On other systems, high-PRF mode may be initiated automatically as the Doppler sample volume is positioned beyond the depth at which spectral aliasing would normally occur. Most systems with this option require the user to first enable the use of auto high-PRF mode through the system setup menu.

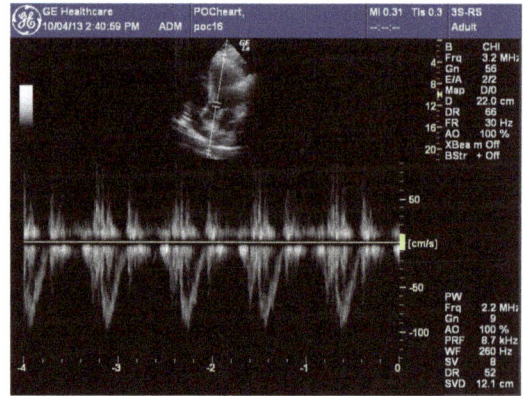

FIGURE 8-12. High-PRF mode pulsed Doppler of the aortic valve. Note the locations of the three sample volumes displayed along the Doppler cursor.

References

Hedrick WR: Technology for diagnostic sonography, St. Louis, 2013, Elsevier.

Hedrick WR, Hykes DL, Starchman DE: Ultrasound physics and instrumentation, ed 4, St. Louis, 2005, Elsevier.

Kremkau FW: Diagnostic ultrasound: principles and instruments, ed 8, Philadelphia, 2011, WB Saunders.

Nichols W, O'Rourke M: McDonalds's blood flow in arteries: theoretical experimental, and clinical principles, ed 5, New York, 2005, Oxford University Press, Inc.

Pellerito J, Polak J: Introduction to vascular sonography, ed 6, Philadelphia, 2012, Elsevier.

9

Basic Scanning Techniques and Ergonomics

OBJECTIVES

- To demonstrate the optimum position for patient, examiner, and equipment to avoid work-related injury.

- To introduce the most common, universally applied transducer manipulation techniques employed during scanning.

KEY TERMS

Anchoring the transducer
Heel-toe manipulation
Negative pressure
Neutral position

Positive pressure
Probe angulation
Probe rotation
Probe translation

INTRODUCTION

Ultrasound scanning is a combination of skill, science, and art. There is a definite set of sonographic techniques that require knowledge and discipline which, when mastered, apply to all areas of scanning. Sonography is unlike other forms of medical imaging in several ways. Primarily, the scanning process is diagnostic in nature, requiring each examination to be customized to the patient in response to observations and

clinical assessment. Unlike radiography or computed tomography, in which rigid protocols are prescribed based on patient history and are not varied during the examination, sonography is adaptable in its execution in response to findings. The sonographer is first an investigator. Information is acquired by exploration, comparison with known normal anatomy and variations thereon, and recognition of abnormal results. Sonography requires a thorough understanding of instrumentation, physics, anatomy, physiology, and the limitations imposed by the combination of these. The knowledge of how to work around these limitations is essential in order to obtain the desired diagnostic information. The examiner must be able to spend as much time as necessary to conduct a comprehensive examination, without strain or fatigue.

Foremost in importance for the sonographer is the development of good habits that minimize strain on the back, arms, wrists, neck, and shoulder joints. A publication issued by the NIOSH in 2006 examined the causes of work-related musculoskeletal injuries in sonographers and included recommendations to help prevent such injuries.[1] The report stated, in part, that injuries resulted from (1) static and awkward postures and movement resulting from the use of the transducer and positioning of both patients and equipment; (2) persistent and continual pressure for sustained periods of time during exams; (3) poor workplace ergonomics in the design of equipment, chairs, tables, and lighting; and (4) increased exam scheduling. Consideration of these factors is even more imperative for users of portable scanners. Most of the larger ultrasound systems have incorporated ergonomic features such as mobility of the monitor and keyboard, devices to assist in cable control, and other equipment designs that are not present on the portable scanners.

Another study by Evans, Roll, and Baker in 2009 surveyed 5200 sonographers and vascular technologists.[2] Of the 2963 who responded, 90% reported that they are currently working in pain. *Shoulder pain is reported as being most common, with older and more experienced sonographers having more finger, hand, and wrist pain than other groups. Pain continues to be related to pressure applied to the transducer, abduction of the arm, and twisting of the neck and trunk.* Ergonomics is an essential component in the practice of ultrasound, both in terms of the long-term health of the sonographer and the ability to conduct the optimal examination.

SCANNING POSITION

Whether a seated or a standing position is utilized by the sonographer, he/she must establish a position where movement and placement of the transducer is controlled absolutely in order to acquire the highest quality diagnostic images. In addition, this scanning posture should be achieved without strain to the sonographer's back, legs, neck, arms, or hands. The goal is for the sonographer's body to be in a neutral position while scanning.

Seated Position

The seated position is always preferable if circumstances permit. A scanning room may be configured to allow sonographers to sit while scanning the patient. Ideally, the height of the scanning table and the chair height are adjustable. Dedicated scanning tables and chairs are not inexpensive, but well worth the extra cost in the form of fewer sonographer injuries and less loss of staff work hours. Chair height and table height are critical in order to enable the sonographer to rest his/her scanning arm upon the patient or some other support (Figure 9-1).

Standing Position

If a standing position is necessary, the table height is the major consideration. Again, the proper table height is critical to allow the sonographer to rest the scanning arm. If the sonographer cannot manage a neutral position and must lean over while scanning, back and shoulder problems will arise.

SCANNING TABLES

In the "old days," obtaining an ultrasound scanning table was simple—just locate a patient litter or stretcher that was not in use. As tempting as that choice may be for the cost-conscious, these devices have been, over the years, a sure formula for sonographer injury. The scanning table should be adjustable in height, be movable, and have lockable wheels. The large bumpers and railings on the sides of patient stretchers prevent a patient from being close to the sonographer. To compensate for the increased separation, the sonographer must bend over to reach the patient. Another poor choice of scanning table is the standard patient exam table found in most physicians' offices. The patient exam table has a fixed height and is difficult for the sonographer to approach closely enough to avoid having to lean and reach. Dedicated

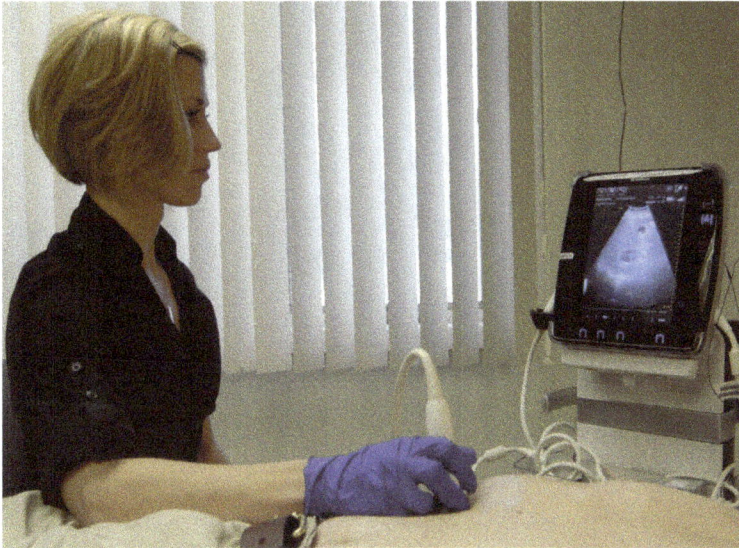

FIGURE 9-1. Seated sonographer with proper chair height and arm support.

scanning tables for various applications as well as adjustable chairs and other ergonomically correct devices are available from a number of manufacturers.

PATIENT POSITION

The sonographer should begin each exam by positioning the patient correctly on the table. The extra few seconds this step requires will be a significant benefit to sonographer in terms of comfort and safety. Positioning or repositioning of the patient must be incorporated into the individual sonographer's workflow to be effective. Moving the patient closer to the examiner by only a few inches can eliminate the need for reaching and bending while scanning (Figures 9-2 and 9-3). Asking a patient to slide an inch or two

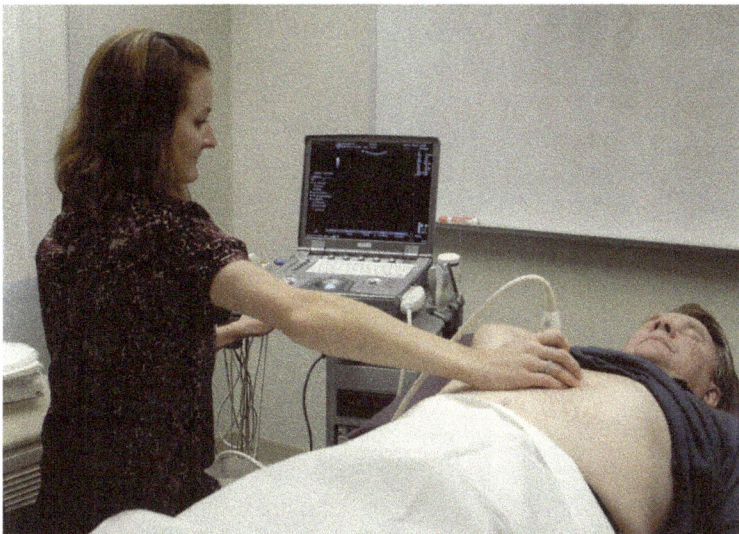

FIGURE 9-2. Seated sonographer in an awkward position having to lean to reach the patient. Observe the absence of arm support.

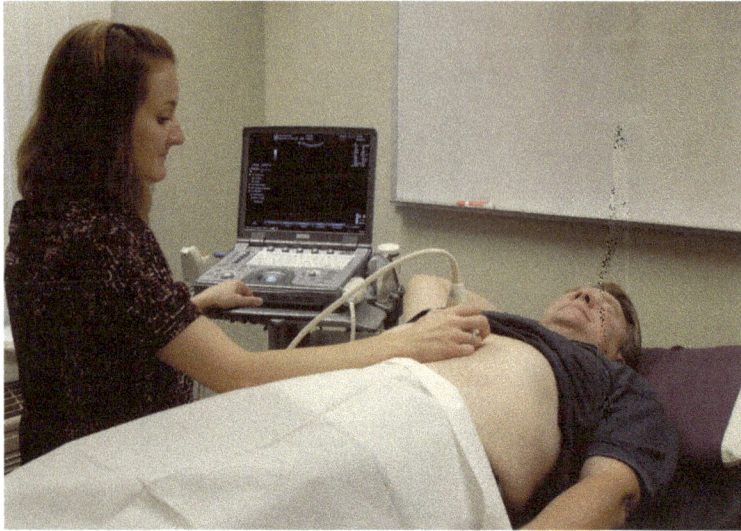

FIGURE 9-3. Patient moved closer to the table edge allowing the sonographer's body and scanning arm to remain in a neutral position with proper arm support.

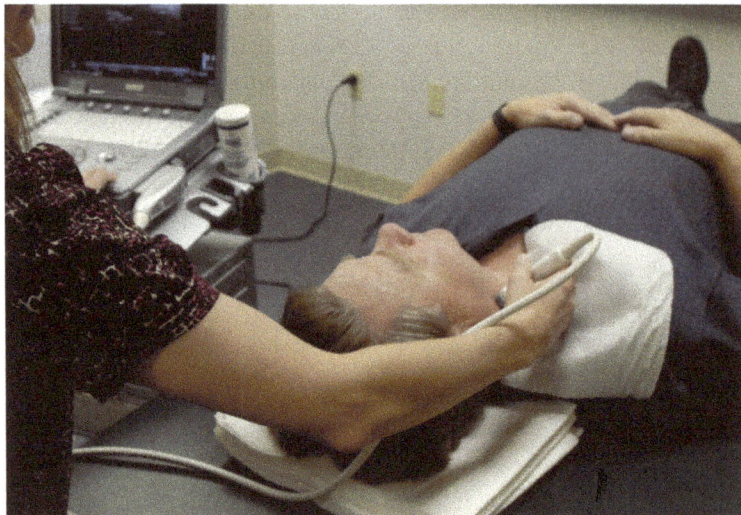

FIGURE 9-4. A carotid scan with patient positioned too far toward the foot of the table causing the sonographer to reach uncomfortably.

toward the head or feet can also positively affect the sonographer's body position (Figures 9-4 and 9-5).

EQUIPMENT SUPPORT PLATFORM

Because portable scanners are easily movable and fold up like a laptop computer, many users assume that they can be placed and operated anywhere there is an available level surface. Portable scanners have been placed on bedside tables, on ECG carts, or next to the patient on the exam table. Sometimes the level surface is formed by holding the device in the lap of the sonographer. All of these are poor choices, both from the point of stability of the instrument and accessibility by the examiner. In addition, care must be taken to provide safe and positive support for the transducer and cable, both of which are

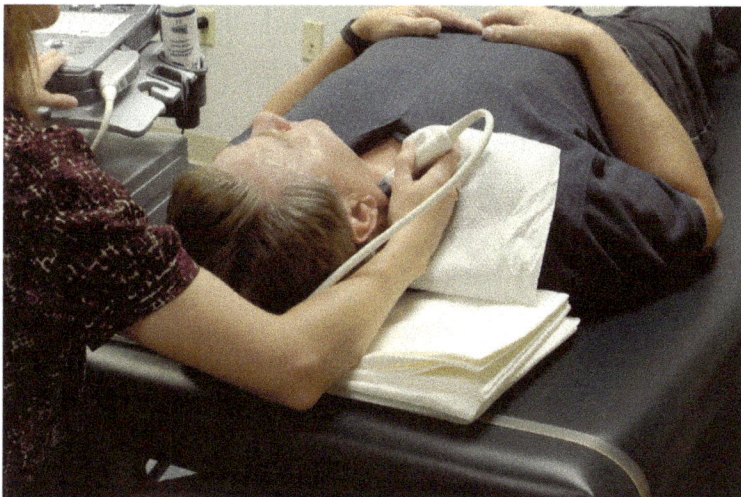

FIGURE 9-5. Patient repositioned a few inches closer to the head of the table with the sonographer's arm now well supported and her body in a neutral position.

susceptible to damage from dropping or pinching. Transducer cables are typically the most vulnerable components of the system. A damaged cable often makes the entire transducer assembly unusable and irreparable. If two or more transducers are available for use with the system, equal care must be taken to protect the transducer(s) that are not currently active, including their cables and connectors. An inadequate platform for the equipment also makes it more difficult for the sonographer to access the system controls and view the monitor without discomfort.

The portable scanner should be adequately supported in a position in which the sonographer is able to operate the controls with his/her free hand (nonscanning hand) without reaching, bending, or twisting. The screen should be positioned such that the sonographer's head is not turned at an acute angle for viewing.

Most manufacturers of mid- to high-end portable units also offer a mobile equipment cart as an option with the system. These carts are typically designed for the specific model of scanner, and most are light enough in weight that they can be picked up and placed into a vehicle trunk or cargo area if the scanner is to be transported to different locations. Although these carts are certainly more expensive than a bedside table, they provide portability, ease of use, and protection of valuable transducers and cables. Figure 9-6 shows examples of portable system carts available from three manufacturers.

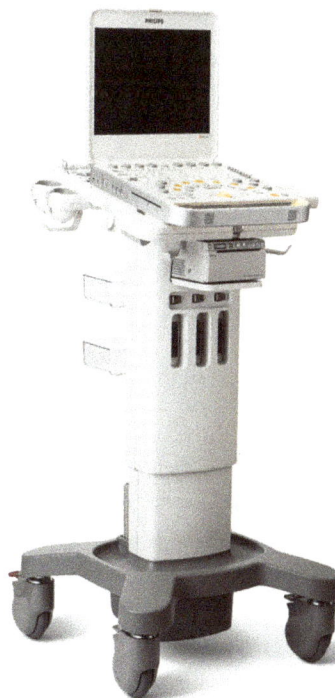

(A)

FIGURE 9-6. Portable equipment carts. (**A**) Philips CX-50 (Courtesy of Philips Healthcare). (*Continued*)

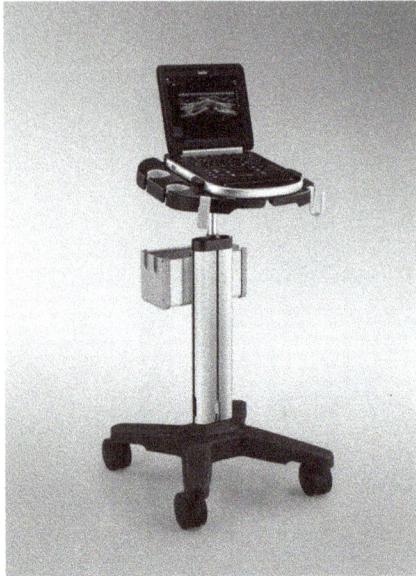

(B)

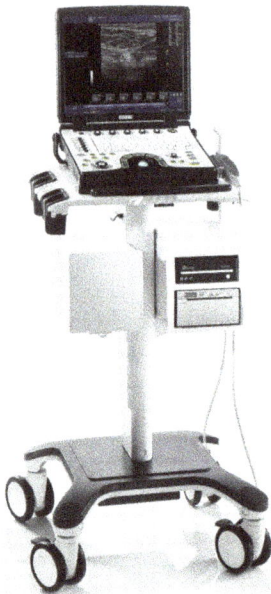

(C)

FIGURE 9-6. (*Continued*) (**B**) Sonosite Edge (Courtesy of FujiFILM-Sonosite, Inc.) (**C**) GE Loqiq-e (Courtesy of GE Healthcare).

EQUIPMENT POSITION

The portable scanner, when adequately supported on a mobile cart, can be repositioned as needed during the course of an ultrasound examination. In order to maintain a neutral posture throughout the examination, especially one like a lower extremity venous evaluation, the sonographer should be able to roll the chair and machine along the table as scanning progresses from the patient's torso region toward the feet. Here again, the mobile equipment cart provided by the manufacturer provides the most flexibility, while assuring adequate protection of transducers and dangling cables (Figure 9-7).

SCANNING ARM SUPPORT

The scanning arm of the sonographer should be supported from the elbow to the wrist if possible. The goal is to create a neutral position for the sonographer's back, neck, arm, wrist, and hand. Neutral position not only protects the operator from injury, but also creates optimal conditions for the sonographer to orient the transducer correctly. Often, the best support option, depending upon the type of examination being performed, is to rest the elbow and forearm on the patient. This option is typically successful for scans of the abdomen, pelvis, adult heart (right-hand technique), and lower extremities. A towel, sheet, or extra paper drapes are placed in such a way that the

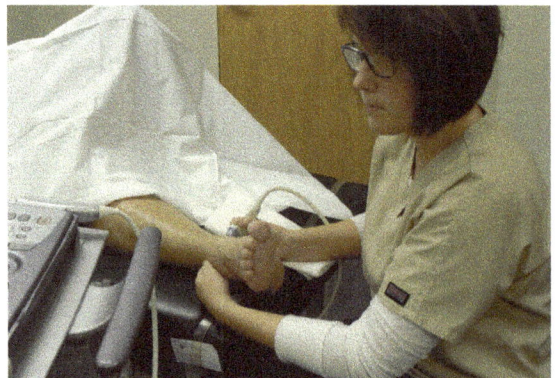

FIGURE 9-7. Seated sonographer performing venous lower extremity exam with machine pulled toward the patient's feet.

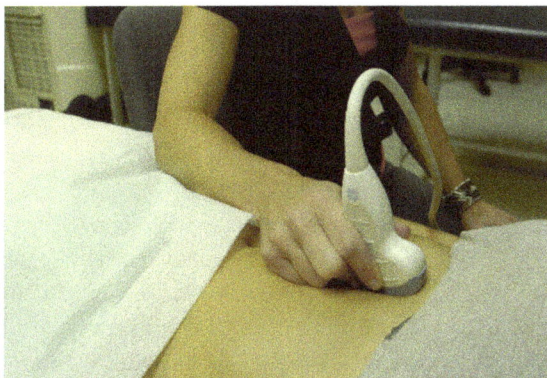

FIGURE 9-8. Seated sonographer performing abdominal exam with drape between scanning arm and patient's skin.

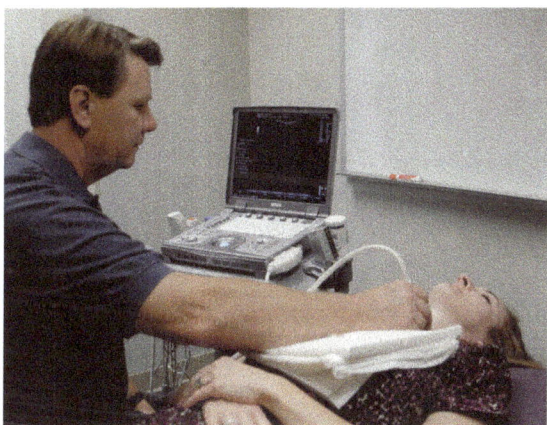

FIGURE 9-9. Sonographer performing thyroid exam with patient drapes placed on patient's upper chest for scanning arm support.

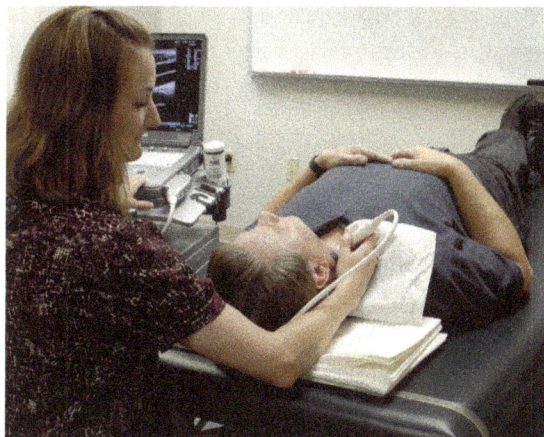

FIGURE 9-10. Sonographer performing a carotid exam with a stack of patient drapes for scanning arm support.

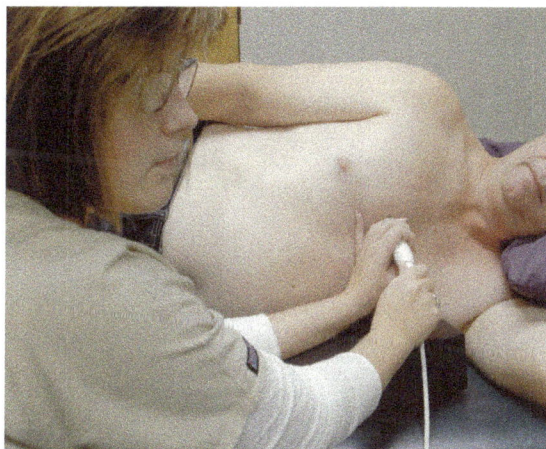

FIGURE 9-11. An echocardiogram performed with the patient lying on his left side, with the sonographer using a foam block to support the scanning arm. Note the use of the opposite hand to stabilize the probe position.

sonographer's arm is not in direct contact with the patient's skin (Figures 9-8 and 9-9).

To establish effective arm support, the heights of the table and chair are of utmost importance. If the chair is too high relative to the table, or if the sonographer is standing and the table is too low, the scanning arm cannot be supported adequately.

In situations where placing the elbow and forearm on the patient's torso is not practical, the sonographer should use folded towels, sponges, wedges, or other devices to support the scanning arm and hand. This is often the case for scanning situations such as the adult heart utilizing the left-hand approach, the shoulder with the patient seated upright, and the

carotid arteries with the examiner seated at the head of the table (Figures 9-10 and 9-11).

When an examination must be performed at the bedside, the sonographer has limited options for optimal table (bed) height as well as body and arm position relative to the patient. Many times in these circumstances the elbow cannot be supported adequately. Therefore, it is critical that the sonographer establish hand and transducer support by implementing optimal transducer grip and anchoring procedure described in the next section. These techniques used to compensate for inadequate arm support are not ideal, however, adequate images may be safely obtained if scanning is completed relatively quickly.

TRANSDUCER GRIP AND HAND SUPPORT

Proper grip of the transducer is essential for the effective manipulation of the transducer. The initial impulse of beginning scanners is often to grasp the transducer very tightly. A tight, rigid grip on the transducer not only defeats the ability to perform most of the basic transducer maneuvers used in scanning, but is also likely to ultimately cause sonographer injuries such as tendonitis and carpal tunnel syndrome.

The transducer should be held with a relaxed, comfortable grip such as one would hold a pencil or a paintbrush. It should be cradled in the palm in such a way as to allow fingertip contact with the patient's skin and control of the probe position with the hand and fingers. The proper grip enables the sonographer to easily manipulate the probe for the various maneuvers described in the following sections. Figure 9-12A shows the transducer cradled in the sonographer's open palm, then the fingers gently encircling the transducer (Figure 9-12B), allowing fingertip control of transducer movements. An incorrectly held transducer does not allow for adequate control (Figure 9-12C). Figure 9-13 demonstrates two examples of a comfortable, well-supported transducer grip.

"Anchoring" the Transducer

One of the most important scanning disciplines is to hold the transducer perfectly still without sliding

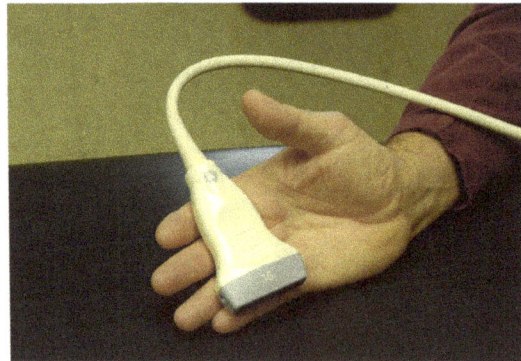

(A)

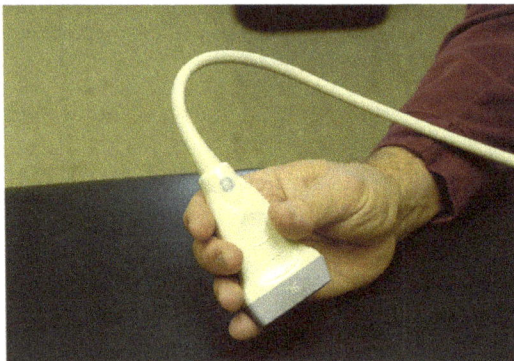

(B)

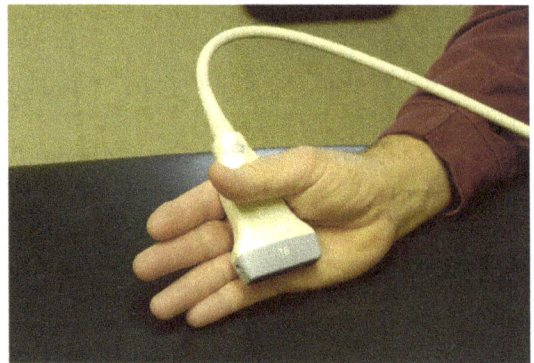

(C)

FIGURE 9-12. (**A**) Probe resting in the open hand. (**B**) Fingers wrapped comfortably around the probe. (**C**) Probe held incorrectly with no fingertip control.

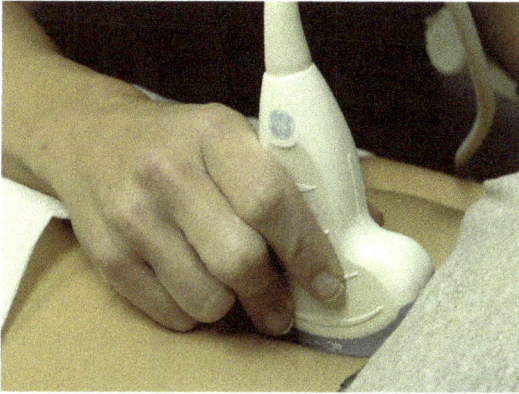

(A)

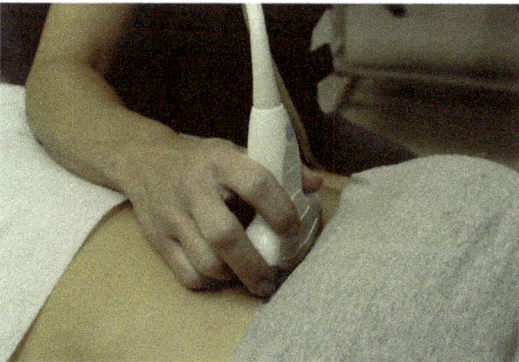

(B)

FIGURE 9-13. (**A**) Probe held in sagittal position. (**B**) Probe held in transverse position. Note the fingertip control of the transducer and the position of the sonographer's fingers in contact with the patient.

to one side or the other. In order to achieve this, the transducer hand must place the probe on the patient's skin surface in such a way that does not cause strain or fatigue to the sonographer's arm and hand, but at the same time allows total control over the transducer position and movement. This is called anchoring the transducer. A common fault of beginning sonographers is that they tend to move the probe constantly while searching for specific anatomical landmarks. The sonographer must realize that scanning is a process that involves establishing the probe position carefully based on external landmarks, and then identifying anatomy while holding the probe still. When probe position must be adjusted, it should be done deliberately and methodically, with movement in

very small increments. Following each movement, the probe must be then held stationary as the examiner considers the anatomy displayed within the image. Effective scanning is a sequence of establishing probe position, readjusting slightly, assessing the image, then re-establishing probe position and reassessing the image, and so forth. The anchor position allows for both stationary scanning as well as controlled movements using any of several manipulation techniques (Figure 9-14A). A probe effectively anchored with the hand and fingers also allows for adequate transducer control even when the examiner and/or the patient is not in an ideal position for resting the arm and wrist, such as when performing studies at the bedside or utilizing an upright patient position (Figure 9-14B).

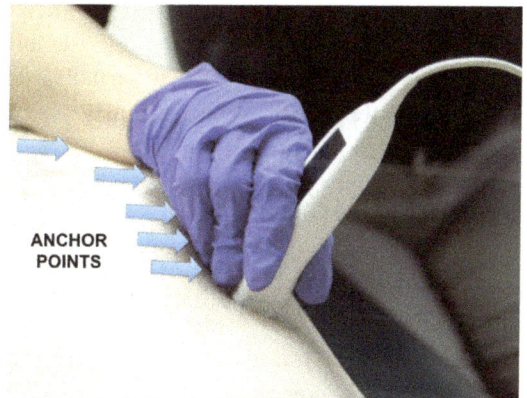

ANCHOR POINTS

(A)

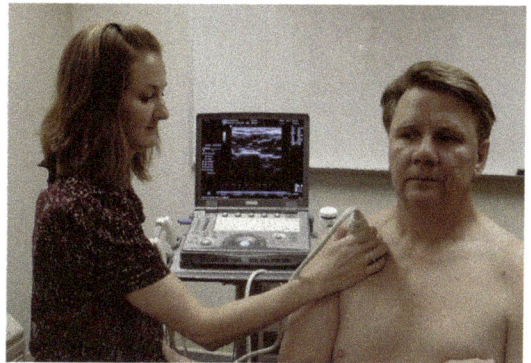

(B)

FIGURE 9-14. Anchoring the transducer. (**A**) Abdominal scan. (**B**) Shoulder scan on an upright patient, probe anchored with the hand and fingers.

TRANSDUCER MANIPULATION TECHNIQUES

Scanning is not simply placing a transducer on the patient and obtaining an image. Rather, a methodical approach involving coordinated transducer movement/position/orientation and adjustment of operator controls is required.

Maintaining Position (Holding Still)

Holding the transducer still in one location is a critical component of diagnostic scanning. The stationary probe enables the sonographer to optimize the image with various operator controls and to systematically identify anatomical landmarks within the field of view. In abdominal scanning, the motionless probe has the added advantage of allowing peristaltic movement within the bowel to possibly open up "windows" to visualize deeply-lying organs (e.g., pancreas) previously obscured by bowel gas.

Two-Hand Approach

The use of the sonographer's opposite hand can often add stability to the probe position and assist in controlling probe movements. In Figure 9-15, two hands stabilize the transducer while scanning intercostally in the abdomen.

Probe Translation

Sliding the transducer to one side or the other, called probe translation, can be a very useful maneuver when following an elongated anatomical structure, or looking for an optimal acoustic window (Figure 9-16).

Angling the Probe

Instead of sliding the transducer, probe angulation, which involves tilting the probe to the left or right at various angles, is often beneficial (Figure 9-17). Angular movement requires the probe footprint to remain fixed, while the probe is tilted. Often, the two

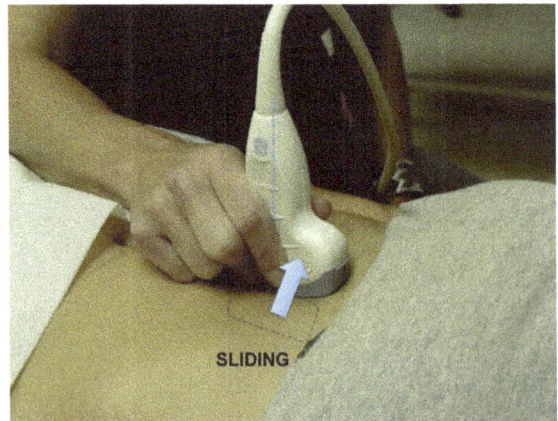

FIGURE 9-16. Translation of probe with arrow showing sliding motion.

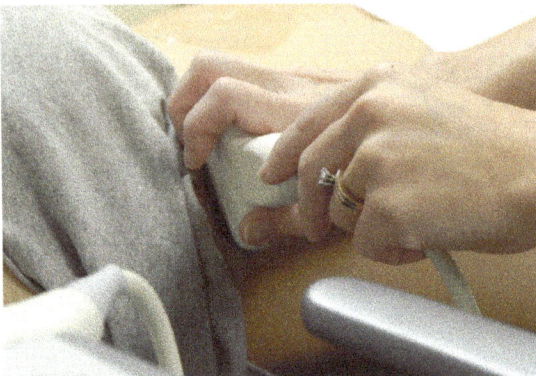

FIGURE 9-15. Probe anchored with two hands for an intercostal scan.

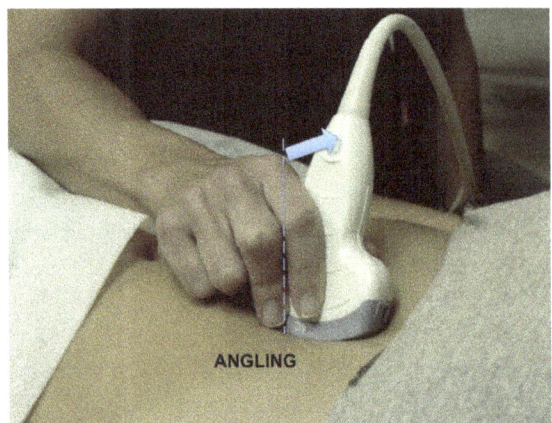

FIGURE 9-17. Tilting the probe with arrow showing angling motion.

motions of translation and angling are combined in sequence, so that the probe is moved very slightly by translation, and then by tilting, and again by sliding. This technique is particularly useful to find the best scanning plane for visualization of the ovaries when performing a female pelvic scan transabdominally.

Probe Rotation

One of the most important transducer maneuvers the beginning scanner must master is the rotation of the probe by 90 degrees about a fixed axis or pivot (Figure 9-18). This technique of probe rotation is applied frequently, whether evaluating blood vessels, abdominal organs, muscles, or ligaments. To execute this maneuver the probe is positioned so that the anatomical structure of interest is placed in the center of the display which then serves as the pivot point. Figure 9-19A shows the common carotid artery in cross section. The probe is then slowly rotated while maintaining the vessel in view, until the vessel is seen in long axis, as shown in Figure 9-19B. As a second example, Figure 9-20A shows the cross-sectional view of the radial nerve, positioned at the center of the image in preparation for 90-degree probe rotation. Figure 9-20B shows the radial nerve in long axis after the 90-degree rotation.

Positive Pressure

Applying positive pressure to the probe is helpful in several situations. Transducer-skin contact can be

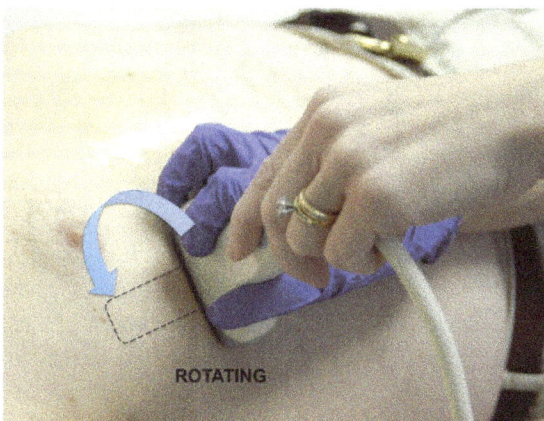

(A)

(B)

FIGURE 9-19. Clinical example of rotation. (**A**) The common carotid artery is visualized in cross section. The probe is then slowly rotated while maintaining the vessel in view. (**B**) At the completion of the rotation the vessel is seen in long axis.

ROTATING

FIGURE 9-18. Technique of 90-degree probe rotation.

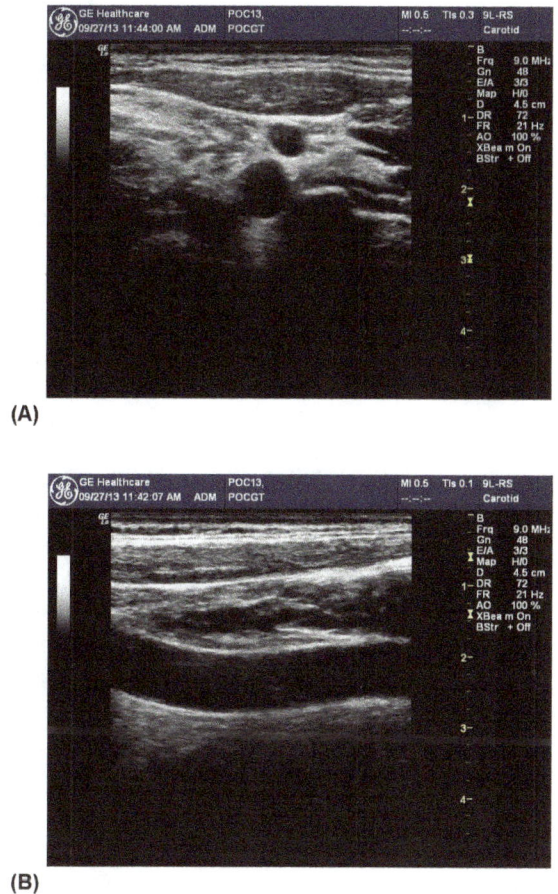

improved and the distance between the transducer and the area of interest can be decreased. Applied over the abdominal region, probe pressure sometimes causes movement of intervening bowel loops, or perhaps the air within the bowel, in order to better visualize organs such as the pancreas or the abdominal aorta. Probe pressure also aids the examiner to differentiate veins from arteries, as most veins will partially or completely collapse due to their low intrinsic pressure. Arteries are compressible but require a much greater probe pressure which is rarely, if ever, indicated.

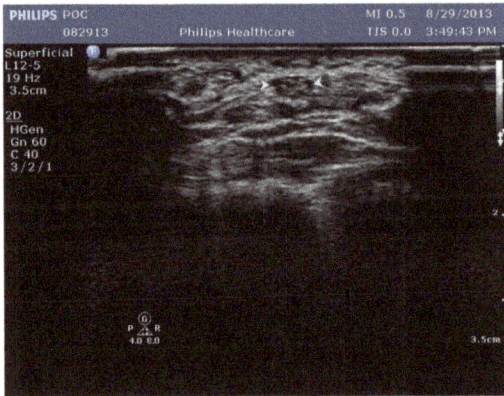

(A)

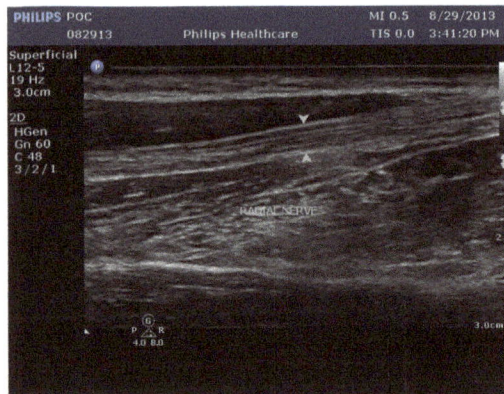

(B)

FIGURE 9-20. Clinical example of rotation. (**A**) Cross-sectional view of the radial nerve, positioned in the center of the image in preparation for 90-degree probe rotation. (**B**) Image of the radial nerve in long axis after the 90-degree rotation (arrows).

Probe compression is one of the two basic tenets of upper and lower extremity venous duplex examinations, and is used to rule out the presence of clot within the vein (Doppler evaluation of the veins is equally important). Figure 9-21 shows positive probe pressure being applied for a femoral vein compression.

Positive Pressure Cautions

In order to avoid hurting the patient, minimal probe pressure should be applied over bony areas, such as ribs or the clavicle, and over superficial organs, such as the thyroid gland. Probe pressure directly over the carotid sinus is inappropriate as it creates the possibility of triggering a vaso-vagal response. However,

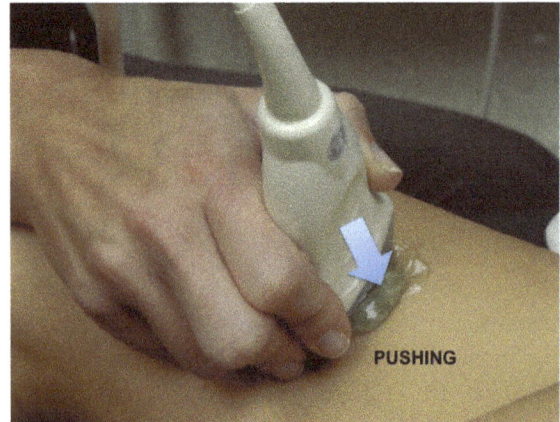

PUSHING

FIGURE 9-21. Positive probe pressure applied for a femoral vein compression.

pressure may be applied during a carotid exam if the probe is placed more laterally over the sternocleido-mastoid muscle. Probe pressure needs to be exercised with discretion in order to prevent musculoskeletal injury to the sonographer. The optimal technique is to apply pressure to the probe carefully and for only a few seconds, just long enough to acquire the desired image. A common reaction of beginning sonographers, when they are having difficulty acquiring an adequate image, is to "push harder." This can quickly become an ingrained habit and is very undesirable from a patient's perspective as well as making sonographer injury much more likely.

Negative Pressure

Negative pressure, in which the probe is supported by the sonographer's hand as it is lifted from the patient's skin, is an extremely useful technique in certain types of examinations and is impossible to achieve without the correct transducer grip and hand position. The key to the application of negative pressure is that the wrist and heel of the hand must be in contact with the patient. The heel of the hand then becomes the fulcrum for the lifting motion of the transducer. This technique is essential for evaluating deep and superficial veins, in particular, as the weight of the probe hand alone will partially or completely collapse many venous structures. Figure 9-22A shows the probe supported with the hand in the normal, or neutral position. As shown in Figure 9-22B,

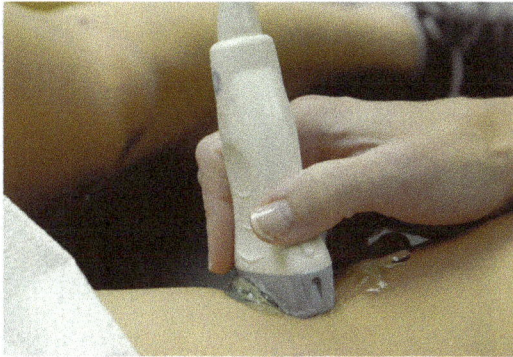

(A)

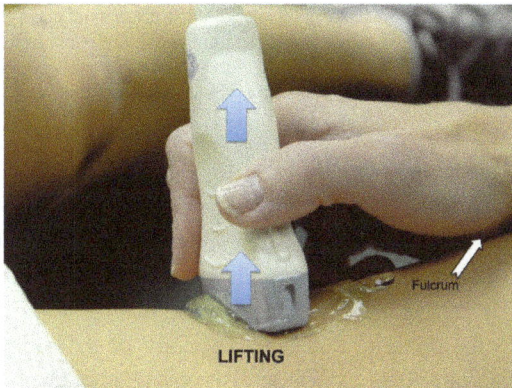

LIFTING

(B)

FIGURE 9-22. Negative probe pressure. (**A**) The probe is supported with the hand in the normal position. (**B**) The hand pivots upward to lift the transducer away from the skin. The heel of the hand acts as the fulcrum (arrows).

the hand pivots upward and the transducer is lifted away from the skin. Acoustic coupling is maintained through the layer of gel. The fifth finger of the scanning hand remains in contact with the skin to ensure probe stability. An ample amount of gel is necessary to eliminate air beneath the transducer face, as the footprint of the probe barely touches the skin. Any superficial structures, especially those located 1 cm or less from the skin surface, are potential candidates to be examined with this technique. By applying a generous amount of gel and lifting the probe, an extra few millimeters of distance between the probe face and the structure of interest may be gained, which is often enough to move the structure of interest beyond the dead zone of the transducer.

Heel-Toe Manipulation

Heel-toe manipulation of the probe is essential to attain an optimal Doppler angle to flow for most blood vessels in the body. Spectral Doppler and color flow evaluation must be performed with the sound beam intersecting the blood flow at an appropriate angle. Ideally, the angle to flow should be 60 degrees or less. The Doppler angle to flow is achieved with a combination of directing the transmitted beam by the Doppler cursor or color box and utilizing the heel-toe technique. In Figure 9-23A, the transducer is shown perpendicular to the skin surface and to the vessel. The resulting image demonstrates poor color filling of the vessel due to the 90-degree angle to flow (Figure 9-23B). By tilting the transducer toward

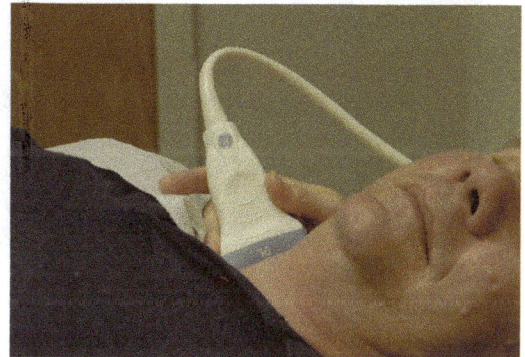

(A)

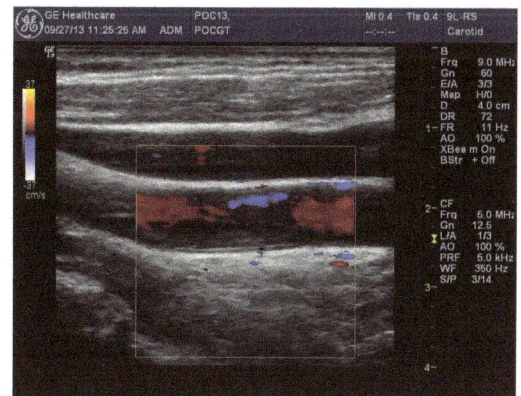

(B)

FIGURE 9-23. Improper Doppler angle to flow. (**A**) The transducer is perpendicular to the skin surface and to the vessel. (**B**) Poor color filling of the vessel due to the 90-degree angle to flow.

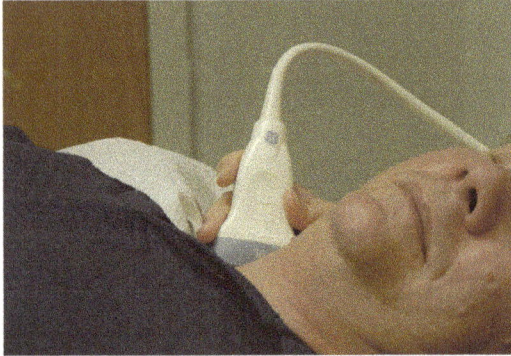

(A)

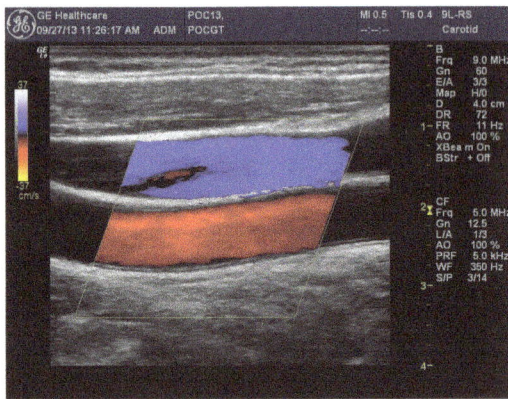

(B)

FIGURE 9-24. Proper Doppler angle to flow. (**A**) The probe is tilted toward the patient's feet utilizing the heel-toe maneuver. (**B**) Excellent color filling of the vessel due to the heel-toe technique and steering of the color box.

the patient's feet utilizing the heel-toe maneuver, the color box is turned in a caudal direction and the resulting image of the common carotid artery now has excellent color filling (Figure 9-24).

When scanning with a curvilinear array or sector transducer, the angle to flow must be accomplished by "swinging" the color box or Doppler cursor to the right or left within the field of view, as the color box is not independently steerable in these transducers (color is restricted to the same scan lines as B-mode). Utilizing the heel-toe technique to position the area to be interrogated on one side or the other of the image usually yields the optimal angle to flow (Figure 9-25).

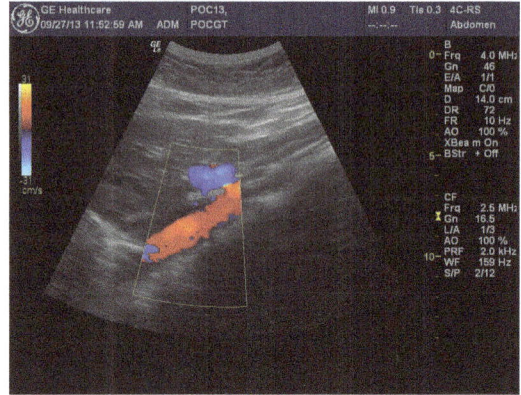

FIGURE 9-25. Color flow image of the abdominal aorta obtained with a curvilinear array transducer. Color angle to flow achieved by the heel-toe technique and swinging the color box toward the left side of the image area.

Cable Support

Even with today's lightweight transducers and cables, the drag and weight of the cable exerts a slight but constant pressure on the transducer that must be counteracted by the sonographer "pulling" the probe in the opposite direction. The force of the cable on the transducer can cause a surprising amount of tension and fatigue in the examiner's hand and forearm (Figure 9-26). Various possible solutions exist, ranging from the sonographer holding the cable in the opposite hand (which unfortunately prohibits the use

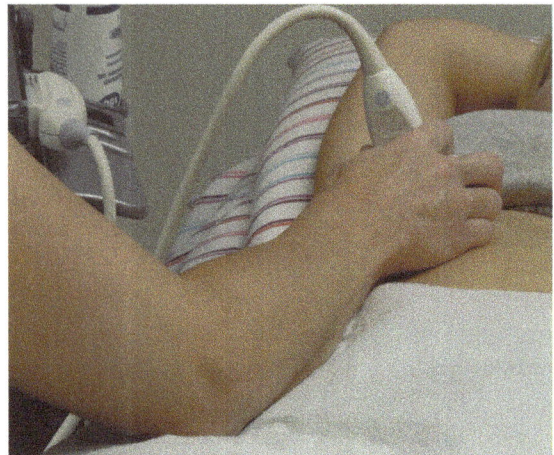

FIGURE 9-26. Cable unsupported exerting constant pressure on probe.

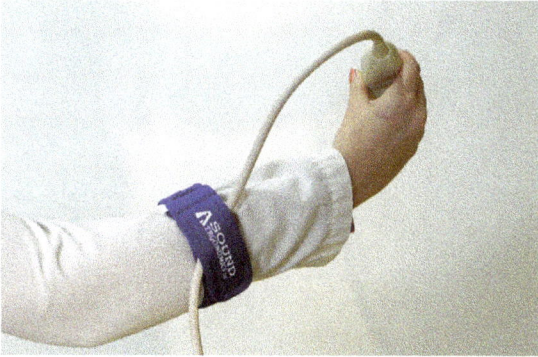

FIGURE 9-27. Cable brace (Courtesy of Sound Ergonomics, LLC).

of the nonscanning hand for other actions) to securing cable under the examiner's leg, under a sponge or wedge used as an arm support, or to another nearby object.

Several commercially available devices have been created for cable control. One such device is the "Cable Brace," available from Sound Ergonomics, LLC.[3] This device attaches to the sonographer's scanning arm and provides an attachment point for cable control (Figure 9-27).

In conclusion, mastery of these basic techniques empowers the sonographer to obtain high-quality diagnostic images, while encouraging habits that minimize the possibility of musculoskeletal injury from scanning.

References

1. National Institute for Occupational Safety and Health: Preventing work-related musculoskeletal disorders in sonography, Washington, DC, 2006 Sep. DHHS Publication number 2006-148.
2. Evans K, Roll S, Baker J: Work-Related Musculoskeletal Disorders (WRMSD) among Registered Diagnostic Medical Sonographers and Vascular Technologists: A Representative Sample. Journal of Diagnostic Medical Sonography 25, 287–299, 2009.
3. Sound Ergonomics, LLC., 6830 NE Bothell Way, Suite C #236, Kenmore, WA 98028 (soundergonomics.com).

10

Clinical Safety

OBJECTIVES

- To state common intensity descriptors.
- To identify the three interactions by which ultrasound may cause damage.
- To understand the indication of risk quantified by the thermal index and the mechanical index.
- To apply the principle of ALARA during sonography.

KEY TERMS

Cavitation
Duty factor
Intensity
Mechanical index
Power
Pulse average

Pulse repetition period
Spatial average
Spatial peak
Temporal average
Temporal peak
Thermal index

MEASUREMENT OF INTENSITY

Intensity is the physical parameter that describes the rate at which energy is conveyed by ultrasound through a small area. Each point within the ultrasonic field has an instantaneous intensity that varies with time (as the wave passes through the region). The potential for biological effects is associated with intensity. High-intensity ultrasound, causing extensive

mechanical distortion, is considered more disruptive to living systems than low-intensity ultrasound. Intensity, by quantifying the temporal and spatial distribution of acoustic energy, provides the most complete description of exposure. A closely related parameter is power, which is the rate of total energy transmission and equals the collected intensity summed over the cross-sectional area of the beam. Traditionally, power is expressed in units of milliwatts (mW) and acoustic intensity in watts per centimeter squared (W/cm^2) or milliwatts per centimeter squared (mW/cm^2).

By placing the transducer in contact with the patient during scanning, acoustic energy is transmitted into tissue. Scanners operate in five different modes—B-mode, M-mode, continuous-wave Doppler, pulsed-wave (PW) Doppler, and Doppler imaging—in which the acoustic output varies over a large range. The highest power is exhibited in color flow imaging and pulsed wave Doppler. Power levels for the same type of device among manufacturers can differ considerably. During linear propagation, frequency, wavelength, and acoustic velocity of an ultrasonic beam are not affected by a change in intensity. However, for high-intensity applications, such as tissue harmonic imaging, propagation is nonlinear and the sinusoidal wave becomes distorted.

Peak negative pressure of a pulsed wave is an important parameter in the consideration of potential damage. The peak negative pressure is also called the peak rarefactional pressure (Figure 10-1). Ultrasound instruments produce peak pressure amplitudes ranging from 0.5 to 5.5 megapascals (more than 50 times greater than atmospheric pressure).

Intensity is proportional to the square of the acoustic pressure. The instantaneous intensity is calculated from the measurement of acoustic pressure in which the acoustic velocity and the density of the medium are known. Unfortunately, acoustic pressure in tissue cannot be measured directly. Typically, the transducer output is quantified using free-field conditions in which a hydrophone placed in water measures the acoustic pressure. The small physical dimension of the hydrophone (0.5–1 mm in diameter) samples a very small area to minimize spatial averaging. The ultrasound wave incident on the hydrophone induces a voltage via piezoelectric effect that is directly proportional to the acoustic pressure. Because the pressure is not constant but fluctuates as the wave passes a point in space, a time-varying waveform of the voltage and thus intensity is obtained. The spatial distribution of intensity is mapped by moving the hydrophone to different locations in the ultrasonic field. Since the attenuation rate for tissue is much greater than that for water, a correction factor (dependent on distance from the transducer) must be applied to convert the free-field intensity to the estimated intensity in tissue.

INTENSITY DESCRIPTORS

Scanning with a pulsed, focused ultrasound beam produces complex spatial and time-varying acoustic fields. Quantification of these patterns for all transducers is impractical and also this detailed information is extremely difficult to correlate with potential bioeffects. Thus, characterization of the ultrasonic field is accomplished by a few select parameters, usually related to energy, such as acoustic power, intensity, or peak negative pressure. The spatial and temporal dependence of the intensity are most often expressed in a simplified form by these shorthand descriptors.

Temporal Dependence

Large fluctuations of intensity are induced in the region through which the sound moves. Each pulsed wave consists of multiple cycles that produce intensity variations within the pulse itself—the maximum intensity designated temporal peak (TP), the intensity averaged over the duration of a single pulse designated pulse average (PA), and the intensity averaged over the longer interval of the pulse repetition period designated temporal average (TA). The pulse repetition period is the total time for one transmission-reception

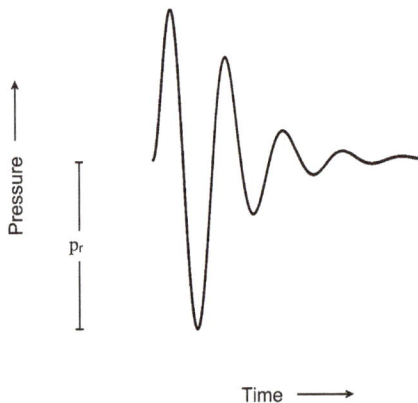

FIGURE 10-1. Pressure variation of a pulsed wave. The peak rarefactional pressure is designated p_r.

cycle, measured from the onset of one transmitted pulse to the onset of the next transmitted pulse. For a given pulse sequence temporal peak has the highest value, followed by pulse average, and finally by temporal average (Figure 10-2).

The temporal-average intensity is considerably smaller than the pulse-average intensity. The ratio of pulse average to temporal average is the duty factor, the fraction of time the transducer is actively generating ultrasound energy. For example, if the pulse duration is 1 μs and the time between pulses is 1 ms, the duty factor is 0.001. The temporal-average intensity is 1000 times less than the pulse-average intensity. A determination of the temporal peak intensity from the pulse-average intensity requires knowledge of the pulse shape. Temporal peak intensity is typically greater than the pulse-average intensity by a factor of 2–10.

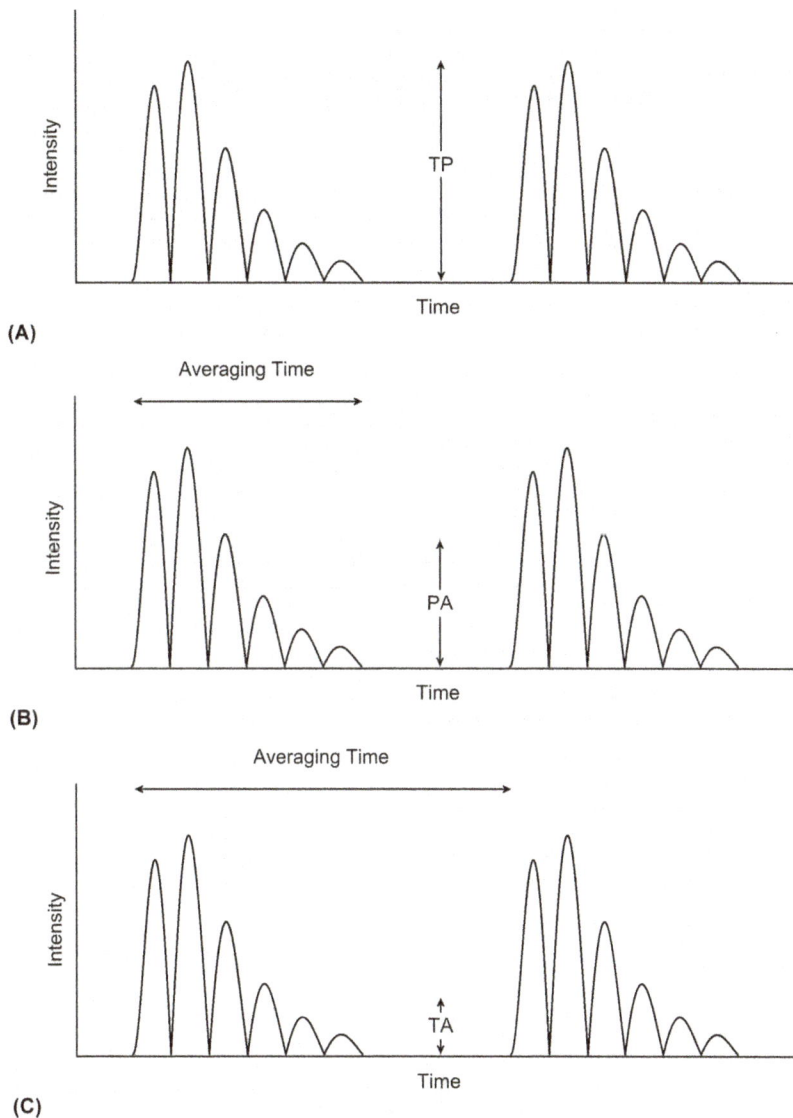

FIGURE 10-2. Specification of intensity with respect to time. (**A**) Temporal peak (TP). (**B**) Pulse average (PA). (**C**) Temporal average (TA).

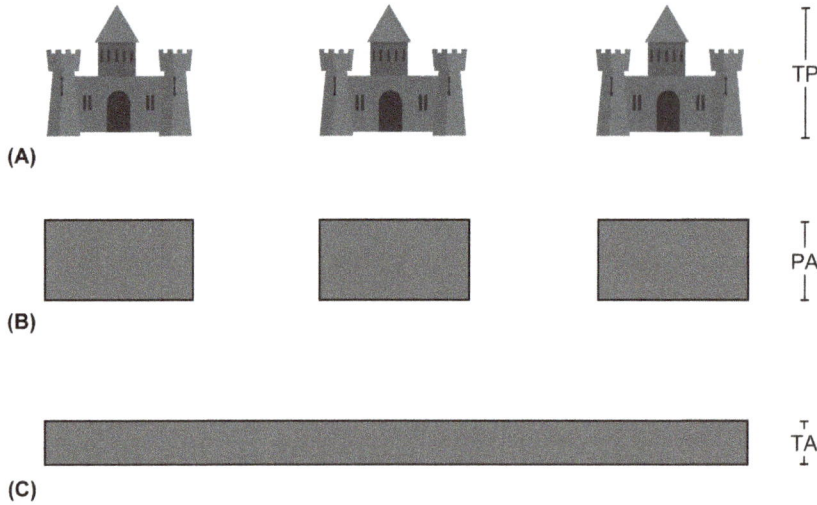

FIGURE 10-3. Temporal averaging. (**A**) The highest points on the sand castles (turrets) correspond to the temporal peak (TP). (**B**) Sand making up the turrets has been flattened and distributed across the base of each castle. This corresponds to the pulse average (PA). (**C**) The sand has been flattened to cover the area between the castles. This corresponds to the temporal average (TA).

The following analogy may help illustrate the relationship between intensity peak and intensity averaging: Suppose a row of sand castles has been built along the seashore, as shown in Figure 10-3. Each castle corresponds to a single pulse. The distance between castles denotes the pulse repetition period. The height of the tallest point of a castle represents the temporal peak. If a castle is flattened so the sand is spread evenly over its base, the level of the sand will be lower than the original peak. This flattened area corresponds to the pulse average. If the sand is distributed over the space between castles, the height of the sand will be reduced further. This represents the temporal average.

Spatial Dependence

The additional factor of space is now considered in the shorthand description of intensity. Once more, the peak or average value with respect to the variable (in this case space) is analyzed. The temporal peak intensity, pulse-average intensity, or temporal-average intensity is mapped as a function of position within the ultrasonic field.

The maximum intensity of all measured values within the ultrasonic field is designated as the spatial peak (SP). Thus, three combinations are possible depending on which temporal intensity is evaluated:

I(SPTP)—Spatial peak, temporal peak intensity
I(SPPA)—Spatial peak, pulse-average intensity
I(SPTA)—Spatial peak, temporal-average intensity

where each intensity descriptor denoted by capital "I" includes a designation specifying how the acoustic field is characterized. The variation in intensity along the axis of propagation for a focused transducer is illustrated in Figure 10-4. The focusing of

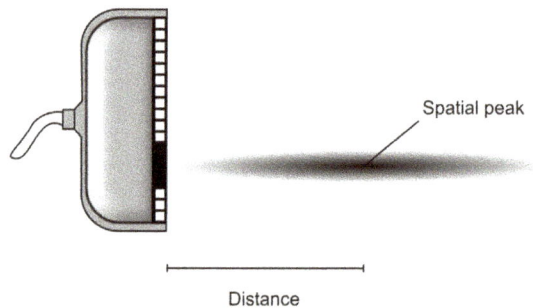

FIGURE 10-4. Intensity variation in the ultrasonic field for a focused transducer. The axial intensity is highest at a particular distance from the face of the transducer, which defines the location and magnitude of the spatial peak intensity.

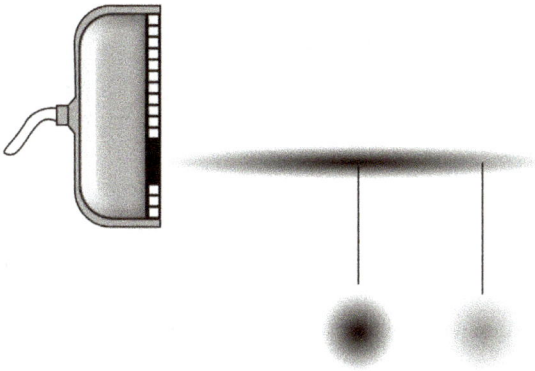

FIGURE 10-5. Relationship of spatial peak (SP) and spatial average (SA) intensities. The intensity variation across the width of the beam is shown for two points. The SA intensity is found by averaging the intensity over the beam cross-sectional area.

the transducer is the most important determinant of the location of the spatial peak.

Spatial averaging (SA) of the temporal intensity over the cross-sectional area of the beam is also a common representation (Figure 10-5). Again, three combinations are possible:

I(SATP)—Spatial average, temporal peak intensity

I(SAPA)—Spatial average, pulse-average intensity

I(SATA)—Spatial average, temporal-average intensity

RISK

The widespread acceptance of ultrasound is attributed in large part to one especially attractive feature—ultrasound is not a type of ionizing radiation. Furthermore, no *acute* harmful effects have been reported following diagnostic ultrasound examinations. Nevertheless, when large populations are exposed to any agent, it is appropriate to investigate any potential long-term effects, which may not be evident on an individual case-by-case basis.

A risk (i.e., potential harmful effect) versus benefit (i.e., diagnostic information derived) analysis is necessary to assess medical efficacy. Quantification of risk from ultrasound examination is not currently available and will never be precisely known. The potential harmful effects to the exposed human population must be inferred from various investigational findings.

A threshold effect is one in which no adverse effect exists below a certain value of a given parameter (in this case, intensity) and above which an adverse and possibly irreversible effect is possible or likely. An illustration of a threshold effect would be the heating of an egg in a skillet. At room temperature the egg white exists as a clear, gelatinous substance. When the temperature of the skillet reaches a certain temperature (the threshold), the protein of the egg white is permanently denatured. In a biological system, intensity levels below a certain value may be incapable of inducing an effect if a threshold exists. For a biologic response with a threshold, adverse effects reported for high intensity are not present at intensity levels lower than the threshold. If the biologic response has no threshold, however, any exposure to the physical agent carries some risk; the question then becomes whether effects observed at high intensity can accurately predict the risk at low intensity based on theoretical models.

For the study of any potential effect, as the probability of that effect approaches zero, the number of individuals necessary to quantify this probability approaches infinity. In most situations, we attempt to avoid large risks and accept risks that may be nonzero but that are too small to measure accurately.

MECHANISMS OF BIOLOGIC DAMAGE

Three mechanisms by which ultrasound interacts with matter have been identified: acoustic radiation force, thermal, and cavitation. Cavitation and radiation force are often classified together as mechanical or nonthermal interactions.

Radiation Force

Radiation force describes damage caused by mechanical vibrations of tissue and generally includes all but thermal and cavitational effects. As the ultrasound wave propagates through the medium by interactions between neighboring particles, the particles undergo considerable changes in velocity and acceleration. An object with a density different from that of the surrounding medium experiences a force in the ultrasound field, because acoustic pressure is applied over its surface. This causes translational or rotational motion of the object. The rotational motion may give rise to acoustic streaming (i.e., circulatory flow of the fluid), and spinning of intracellular particles may be induced. At high intensities, high-velocity gradients are formed near solid boundaries. The resulting microstreaming (i.e., rapid movement of fluid in a localized area) can fragment the macromolecules in these regions. This generally occurs at intensity levels much greater than diagnostic ultrasound and is not of concern in clinical practice.

Thermal Interactions

As the ultrasound beam propagates through tissue, acoustic energy is converted into heat. The increased temperature has the potential to cause irreversible tissue damage. Time at elevated temperature necessary to elicit a response, particularly for the fetus, is well documented. The rate of temperature rise depends on the temporal-average intensity, the rate of absorption, the cross-sectional area of the beam, the duration of exposure, and the heat-transport processes (thermal conductivity and blood flow). Within the frequency range of 1–20 MHz, the rate of energy absorption increases with frequency. Thermal effects dominate at the low megahertz frequencies and tend to mask other (nonthermal) effects.

Cavitation

Regions of compression and rarefaction are created along the path of propagation. Tissue is subjected to increases and decreases in pressure in an alternating fashion, and these pressure fluctuations cause gas bubbles to exhibit dynamic behavior. The gas bubbles may preexist in tissue or may be formed by the wave action. This phenomenon is known as cavitation, which can be either stable or transient.

STABLE CAVITATION

In stable cavitation, microbubbles already present in the medium expand and contract during each cycle in response to the applied pressure. The bubbles may also grow as dissolved gas leaves the solution during the negative-pressure phase. Each bubble oscillates about the expanding radius for many cycles without collapsing completely. At a specific frequency of sound, dependent on the microbubble size, the vibration amplitude is maximized.

The action of the gas bubble in the liquid is analogous to a child's swinging on a swing. An external force (push) applied to the child at the proper instant in the oscillatory path increases the height of the swing. If the force is repeated over and over at the proper frequency, the motion of the swing is amplified. If the child is pushed opposite the direction of movement, the height of the swing decreases. The interplay between the rate of pushing and the physical characteristic of the swing (e.g., length of rope between the pivot point and the seat) is essential for maximum effect. Similarly, in cavitation, the interaction between the size of the gas bubble and the frequency becomes critically important.

A free air bubble in water undergoes resonance at 1 MHz when its radius is 3.5 microns. At higher frequencies, the size of the bubble required for resonance decreases. Bubbles somewhat smaller than resonance size tend to grow, whereas those significantly larger than resonance size do not sustain stable cavitation. Oscillations of a gas bubble may produce high shearing forces in the nearby surrounding areas. Stable cavitation may also give rise to microstreaming. The radial oscillatory motion of the bubble is not always spherically symmetrical. An adjoining solid boundary may distort the motion of the bubble and cause eddies near the gas-liquid interface. High-velocity gradients are created in the localized region of the oscillatory boundary layer. Biomolecules or membranes subjected to such gradients can fragment or rupture.

TRANSIENT CAVITATION

Transient cavitation is a more violent form of microbubble dynamics in which short-lived bubbles undergo large changes in size over a few acoustic cycles before collapsing completely. Bubbles of submicron dimensions may already be present in the medium or may be formed by dissolved gases leaving the solution during the rarefaction phase. Bubble growth also takes place during the rarefaction phase, which is enhanced by low-pressure periods of long duration. That is, low-frequency sound is more likely to exhibit transient cavitation. High viscosity and surface tension inhibit bubble growth.

During the compression phase, increased pressure causes the bubbles to collapse and produce highly localized shock waves. In addition, very high temperatures and pressures are created within the bubbles, resulting in the decomposition of water into free radicals. These pressures and temperature changes may also drive chemical reactions.

The general consensus is that transient cavitation is a threshold effect. The peak negative pressure necessary to cause cavitation increases with frequency, exhibiting a square root of frequency dependence. This means that sound intensity just sufficient to cause cavitation at low frequency does not initiate cavitation at higher frequency. Transient cavitation has been demonstrated in mammalian systems at pressure levels generated by diagnostic imaging equipment. However, gas bodies or bubbles must be present for cavitation to occur. Further, cavitation is limited to a small area affecting very few cells, which makes detection of damage very difficult. Exposure to the lung and intestine can produce small, localized hemorrhages in laboratory animals, but appear to resolve naturally and without lasting effects in healthy subjects. In the absence of gas bodies no biologically significant adverse effects related to cavitation have been demonstrated at diagnostic pressure and frequency levels.

EPIDEMIOLOGIC STUDIES

Although animal research has provided some insight into and reassurance regarding the potential harm from ultrasound exposure at diagnostic levels, the application of these data to human populations is limited. The ultimate assessment of biologic effects induced in human populations exposed to ultrasound is derived from epidemiologic studies. This type of investigation attempts to answer the question whether individuals exposed to a particular agent have a higher risk of developing impaired health than nonexposed individuals do. The ideal study design identifies two groups in which the only difference between groups is exposure history to the agent. If the additional risk to an exposed population is small, a large number of individuals must be studied to distinguish the agent-induced effects from disorders that occur spontaneously. A long latent period (i.e., the delay between exposure and observable effect) necessitates that these populations are monitored over a period of many years. Collecting data for a large population over a long time is an extremely expensive undertaking and subject to error. The agent of interest is most likely not the only cause of a health disorder; furthermore, the risk of an induced effect is not the same for all members of the population.

Rarely does a single study become the definitive work regarding identification of an adverse effect and related risk factors from exposure to a particular agent. The overall assessment is based on multiple, imperfect studies conducted under diverse conditions involving different populations. Epidemiologic studies are often flawed either in experimental design or by incompleteness of the data. To establish an agent as the potential cause, a consistent pattern must develop whereby the results from different studies associate the same biologic effect(s) with prior exposure to the agent, produce rate of occurrence dependent on the amount of agent exposed, and demonstrate a similar time sequence with respect to onset of the adverse effect.

Low birth weight, fetal chromosome abnormalities, structural fetal anomalies, altered neurologic development, cancer, and hearing disorders have been investigated as possible adverse effects from fetal exposure to ultrasound. No association between in utero ultrasound exposure and fetal chromosome abnormalities, congenital malformations, cancer, and hearing disorders has been demonstrated. Several studies, including three randomized clinical trials, have found no association between low birth weight and in utero exposure. The finding of reduced birth weight in two retrospective studies has little clinical importance. Suggestions of delayed speech and abnormal reflexes from in utero exposure in isolated surveys are not generally supported by multiple studies that show negative findings.

Results of the epidemiologic studies have been generally negative, which indicates that damage, if any, is subtle, delayed, or infrequent. The number of subjects in a study reporting negative results places an upper limit on the incidence rate of an adverse effect, but it does not exclude the induction of the effect by ultrasound. For those studies with positive findings, the association of ultrasound exposure with a particular outcome does not absolutely establish ultrasound as the causative agent. The association may be the result of shared underlying factors or statistical variations. Various scientific organizations have concluded that a causal relationship between diagnostic ultrasound and adverse effects has not been demonstrated by the congregated epidemiologic studies conducted to date.

RISK VERSUS BENEFIT

Although harmful effects of ultrasound have not been demonstrated after exposure at diagnostic levels, the data are not sufficient to permit unquestioned acceptance of its safety. The risk is extremely low but may not be zero. During a diagnostic ultrasound examination energy is directed into the patient, which perturbs the biological system and may ultimately create some risk, albeit small, of causing damage. The prudent course of action therefore is to apply objective criteria in the selection of patients for an ultrasound examination and to practice the principle of ALARA (as low as reasonably achievable). The application of ALARA means the operator optimizes the diagnostic information content while minimizing exposure. In other words, the benefit must outweigh the risk. Exposure in this sense consists of acoustic output (power, intensity, or peak pressure) and duration of scanning. *Education, training, and experience of the operator have a major effect on exposure, both power levels and examination times.*

A diagnostic ultrasound examination should be conducted only when medically indicated. *Medically indicated* implies that some benefit can be expected from the information obtained. Furthermore, a power level consistent with the objectives of the examination should be used. A low power setting that does not provide the desired diagnostic information exposes the patient unnecessarily. Although the exposure is low, no benefit is gained. The same principles apply to an examination so limited in time as to compromise the validity of the study.

THERMAL CONSIDERATIONS

For life processes to be maintained, the body temperature must stay within a narrow range. Although a variation of 1°C is tolerable (and indeed common), thermal-mediated fetal abnormalities can result from temperature elevation. *Avoiding a local rise in temperature above 1°C should ensure that no biologic effects are induced.*

Acoustic energy is converted to heat as the ultrasound beam passes through tissue. The rate of heating depends on the time-averaged intensity, the absorption properties of the tissue (bone absorbs sound energy more efficiently than soft tissue), beam width, and the frequency. The rate of absorption for most tissues increases linearly with frequency. Focused beams, by creating ultrasonic fields with nonuniform intensity, can cause small, localized regions of heating. The removal of heat from small volumes (narrow beam width and short focal zone) is very rapid. Continuous insonation ultimately produces a steady state condition in which the maximum temperature does not change.

Temperature Profiles

Temperature profiles along the axis of a focused beam can be calculated for a given set of conditions using various tissue models: presence or absence of bone, absorption properties of tissues, transducer aperture, focal length, frequency, power, and degree of perfusion. Sound energy is readily transferred to bone. Figure 10-6 illustrates the effect on heating for the placement of the focal zone relative to bone. As frequency is increased, absorption by all tissues is also increased. If the same amount of energy is deposited over an increasingly wide area (controlled by aperture and beam scanning), then resulting

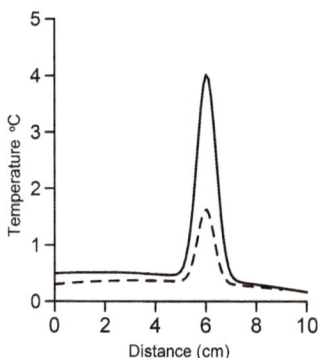

FIGURE 10-6. Temperature profiles along the axis for transmit focused length of 6 cm (solid line) and 10 cm (dotted line) using a model in which fetal bone is located at a depth of 6 cm. Bone within the focal zone elevates heating.

temperature rise is less. The induced maximum temperature does not occur instantaneously, but rather requires some duration of exposure to achieve this condition (a pot of water placed on the hot stove does not boil immediately).

OUTPUT DISPLAY STANDARD

In 1992, the American Institute of Ultrasound in Medicine and the National Electrical Manufacturers Association adopted the voluntary standard for display of acoustical output information called the Output Display Standard. Two acoustic output parameters, the thermal index (TI) and the mechanical index (MI), are defined as indicators of the potential for biologic effects. The thermal index, in essence, gives the maximum temperature rise in tissue that can be predicted from sonographic examination, and the mechanical index describes the likelihood of cavitation.

The output indices are displayed in real time for the selected scanner parameters for immediate feedback to the operator. The operator controls of transmit power, frequency, and focusing affect the mechanical index. The thermal index depends on the temporal-average intensity, pulse repetition frequency (scan range and frame rate), and frequency. Receiver controls including gain, time gain compensation, gray-scale mapping, dynamic range, and image processing have no effect on these indices.

Determining acoustic intensity distributions along various tissue paths for diverse equipment and operating modes in use today is not possible. Thermal and mechanical indices are generated from simplified models using conservative worst-case conditions. The indices provide a uniform basis for the assessment of risk. Since acoustic output information is standardized, operators can implement the same safety principles to all diagnostic ultrasound equipment regardless of manufacturer.

THERMAL INDEX

Temperature elevation depends on power, frequency, transducer aperture, tissue types, beam dimensions, and scanning mode. Scanned mode or autoscanning refers to the sweeping or steering of successive transmitted pulses through the field of view. In scanned modes, such as B-mode, the sound energy does not pass through the same area repeatedly, but instead the transmitted pulse is directed along the next adjacent line of sight, thus spreading the energy over a larger volume. In non-scanned modes, such as M-mode or spectral Doppler, the same line of sight is sampled repeatedly, thereby concentrating the energy in one location. Tissue heating may occur more rapidly in the non-scanned mode. Ultimately, the amount of heating is governed by energy transfer to tissue and the volume over which that absorbed energy is distributed. Operator controls that increase power output will increase the thermal index.

Three thermal indices corresponding to soft tissue (TIS), bone (TIB), and cranial bone (TIC) have been developed depending on whether bone is encountered along the path, and if it is, whether bone is located near the transducer or in the interior of the body. TIS applies when the beam path consists of soft tissue only and bone is not present (examinations of the abdomen and fetus during the first trimester). The highest temperature rise occurs near the surface where the B-mode beam enters the patient. In PW Doppler and M-mode, transmit pulses are directed along a single scan line (non-scanned mode) and the highest temperature rise is between the surface and the focal zone. If bone is encountered near the transducer, then TIC is used (examinations of pediatric and adult head). TIB applies if the ultrasound beam, after passing through soft tissue, impinges on bone near the focal zone (examinations of the fetus during the second and third trimesters).

The thermal index is defined as the ratio of the scanning power level to a reference value, which is calculated using a specific tissue model and operating parameters. The reference value is the best estimate of the power that would cause a 1°C temperature rise at some point within the ultrasonic field. By comparing the output power to this reference value, *thermal index predicts the temperature rise in °C for the selected operator controls*. If the output power is equal to the reference value, the thermal index is 1. If the output power is twice the reference value, the thermal index is 2.

Tissue type, blood perfusion, presence of fluid, and exposure time may not be accurately characterized by the model causing the actual patient temperature to deviate from that predicted by the thermal index. The scanning time is often less than the time required to reach steady state, and in that circumstance, the thermal index overestimates the temperature rise in tissue. For poorly perfused tissue in contact with the transducer or the presence of fluid along the sound path, the temperature rise may be higher than that predicted by the thermal index. If sound path is long (obese patients, large muscular patients, and deep-lying structures), then the thermal index may overestimate the temperature rise. In the circumstance of nonlinear propagation, the thermal index may underestimate temperature rise in tissue at high power levels. Nevertheless, the thermal index does provide the relative effect on tissue heating when operator controls are changed. Adjustment of scanner parameters such that the thermal index increases from 0.5 to 1 indicates that the anticipated temperature rise has doubled.

MECHANICAL INDEX

The pulsed ultrasound wave, consisting of multiple cycles, causes large fluctuations in acoustic pressure as it moves through tissue. Cavitation is more likely to occur at high pressures and low frequencies. The cavitation threshold under optimal conditions with pulsed ultrasound is predicted by the mechanical index, the ratio of the peak negative pressure to the square root of the frequency. Scientific research has indicated that cavitation-induced effects may be possible at peak pressures and frequencies within the operational range of diagnostic equipment. Specifically, lung and intestinal hemorrhages in mice have been reported at diagnostic output levels.

The ultrasonic field is represented by a single value of the mechanical index. This is a conservative assessment based on an assumed low rate of attenuation for tissue (0.3 dB/cm-MHz). The location within the ultrasonic field where cavitation is most likely to occur is unknown to the operator. Along a poorly attenuating path such as when fluid is present or during nonlinear propagation, the displayed mechanical index underestimates the potential for cavitation. For a long sound path the calculated pressure in tissue overestimates the mechanical index.

DISPLAY OF OUTPUT INDICES

Ultrasound equipment, which has the potential to produce an index value above 1, must be able to display that index in real time as operator controls are changed. If the scanning parameters are such that the index value falls below 0.4, then display of the index is not necessary. B-mode scanners are not capable of producing a temperature rise above 1°C, and thus only the mechanical index is displayed during this mode of operation. For other modes, displays of both the mechanical index and thermal index are possible, although not necessarily simultaneously. The mechanical index is displayed during B-mode imaging and the thermal index during PW Doppler, M-mode, and Doppler imaging using the display criteria stated above.

OUTPUT INDICES AS RISK INDICATORS

Thermal index is a conservative estimate based on a worst-case assumptions. Although the calculated temperature in tissue is subject to many uncertainties, an upper limit of the actual temperature rise from typical clinical examinations is inferred. Insonation of long duration is often necessary to achieve the temperature rise predicted by the thermal index. Cavitation is generally believed to be a threshold phenomenon. The presence of gaseous bodies (lung, gastrointestinal tract, contrast agents) makes cavitation more likely.

The acoustic output indices serve as risk indicators. If the index value is below the threshold level for bioeffects (considered 0.5–1), then a further decrease in acoustic output would not improve safety and may compromise the diagnostic information content. At an index value less than 0.5, adverse effects associated with tissue heating and cavitation are considered nonexistent. For higher index values, a judgment of risk versus benefit is necessary. TIBs for commercially available systems range from 0.1 to 10 for fetal scanning. At the highest thermal index values, scanning for more than a few seconds may cause harm.

Practical guidelines using the thermal and output indices have been published by Nelson et al. The prenatal examination should be conducted with a thermal index less than 0.5, if possible. If the thermal index exceeds 2.5, the time should be limited to less than 1 minute and if the thermal index is 0.5–1 the time can be extended to 30 minutes. A mechanical index of less than 0.4 is recommended. For the postnatal examination, a thermal index less than 2 may be used for scanning times on an extended basis. If the thermal index exceeds 6, then the time should be limited to less than 1 minute and if the thermal index is 2–6, then the time can be extended to 30 minutes. A mechanical index of less than 0.4 is recommended, but in the absence of gas bodies may be raised to as high as 1.9, if needed.

AMERICAN INSTITUTE OF ULTRASOUND IN MEDICINE

The American Institute of Ultrasound in Medicine (AIUM) reviews current findings regarding bioeffects and applies this knowledge to the assessment of the risk associated with clinical diagnostic ultrasound. Critiques of research reports and statements regarding the safety of diagnostic ultrasound are published regularly. Its conclusions are acknowledged to be safety guidelines throughout the ultrasound community.

The AIUM has assessed potential bioeffects attributable to ultrasound irradiation of non-human mammalian tissue. No adverse biological effects related to the thermal mechanism have been demonstrated if the spatial peak, temporal average is less than 100 mW/cm^2 for unfocused beams and less than 1 W/cm^2 for focused beams or if the thermal index is less than 2. Higher values of the thermal index do not cause harm if the duration of exposure is regulated: 1 m for thermal index of 6, 10 m for thermal index of 4, and 100 m for thermal index of 2.7. When non-thermal mechanism is considered, no adverse effects are associated with peak rarefactional pressures below 0.3 MPa or mechanical index less than 0.3. These conclusions summarize the research regarding biological effects following ultrasound exposure, but do not provide an absolute level of safety.

The AIUM has also examined the clinical safety of diagnostic ultrasound and has found that in the absence of contrast agents no adverse effects have occurred at intensity levels of FDA-approved devices (spatial peak, temporal-average intensity of 720 mW/cm^2 and mechanical index less than or equal to 1.9). AIUM further concludes that children who were exposed to ultrasound in utero exhibit no adverse effects. The AIUM statement on prudent use considers current aspects of clinical safety:

> Diagnostic ultrasound has been in use since the late 1950s. Given its known benefits and recognized efficacy for medical diagnosis, including use during human pregnancy, the American Institute of Ultrasound in Medicine herein addresses the clinical safety of such use: No independently confirmed adverse effects caused by exposure from present diagnostic ultrasound instruments have been reported in human patients in the absence of contrast agents. Biological effects (such as localized pulmonary bleeding) have been reported in mammalian systems at diagnostically relevant exposures but the clinical significance of such effects is not yet known. Ultrasound should be used by qualified health professionals to provide medical benefit to the patient. Ultrasound exposures during examinations should be as low as reasonably achievable. (ALARA)

A summary of bioeffects, clinical applications demonstrating the prudent use, and techniques to implement ALARA is published in "Medical Ultrasound Safety," second edition, 2009.

CLINICAL EFFICACY

Technical capabilities and clinical applications have advanced dramatically during the past 25 years, such that more than 100 million sonographic examinations are conducted each year within the United States alone. Anatomic detail, high information content, short duration of exams, immediate feedback of results, record of safety, acceptance by patients, ease of use, portability, durability, and relatively low cost have driven this increased utilization of diagnostic ultrasound.

Because ultrasound yields excellent anatomic visualization and is generally considered to be without harmful effects, obstetrics is particularly well suited for this imaging modality. In the United States, approximately 80% of the 4 million children born each year are examined sonographically in utero. Although ultrasound is assumed to contribute to the improved management and outcome of a pregnancy, clinical efficacy for all patients has not been demonstrated. A randomized clinical trial, the Routine Antenatal Diagnostic Imaging with Ultrasound (RADIUS), examined the premise that routine screening reduces perinatal morbidity and mortality. For low-risk populations, this study found that routine screening with ultrasound did not reduce perinatal mortality and morbidity beyond that achieved by selective examination based on clinical judgment. Nevertheless, routine screening with ultrasound for every pregnant patient has become more and more common in the United States and abroad.

Ultrasonography during pregnancy, in addition to providing an assessment of maternal and fetal well-being, may have other less tangible benefits. Viewing the monitor screen with explanation of the images as part of a medically indicated ultrasound examination may improve maternal perception of the fetus and maternal-infant bonding. The maternal attitude can influence fetal outcome by causing prenatal behavioral changes (e.g., cessation of smoking and reduced alcohol consumption). However, ultrasonography during pregnancy should not be performed for the sole purpose of viewing the fetus by the mother or determining its sex. Other commercial demonstrations of ultrasound imaging during pregnancy without medical benefit are inappropriate. Although the risk in these instances is very low, risk will always outweigh benefit where medical or educational benefit is zero.

USER RESPONSIBILITY

Diagnostic ultrasound has well-established medical applications with known benefits and recognized efficacy. Prudent use dictates that objective criteria should be applied in the selection of patients for an ultrasound examination. Furthermore, qualified health professionals should conduct the examination at minimum power levels and scanning time to obtain the desired diagnostic information. The principle of ALARA, when applied, compels the operator to conduct the examination with the lowest reasonable exposure to the patient. The practice of ALARA is facilitated using the real-time, displayed output indices, thermal index and mechanical index. Exposure to the patient should be minimized by adjusting acquisition parameters that contribute to energy deposition in the patient while maintaining the desired information content. Often, the default power level is set at 100% for a given application. However, output power can often be reduced to relatively low levels with no loss of image quality (Figure 10-7). For best practice, the output power should be adjusted to the minimum output required to obtain the desired information. On scanners where the output power is not directly adjustable, correct settings of secondary controls such as display depth and examination preset, along with diligent attention to the output display indices, are essential to maintaining acceptable patient exposure levels. Scanning should be limited to the anatomy of interest. PW Doppler and color Doppler imaging should be utilized when these operational modes contribute significant diagnostic information.

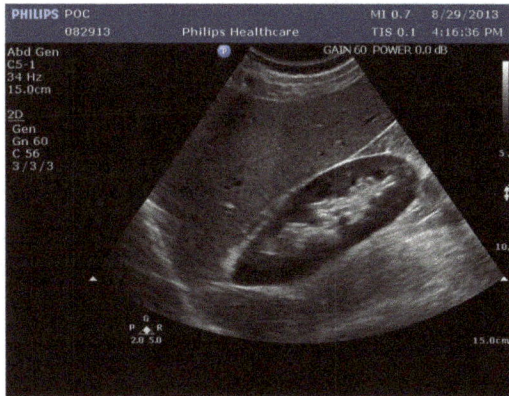

(A)

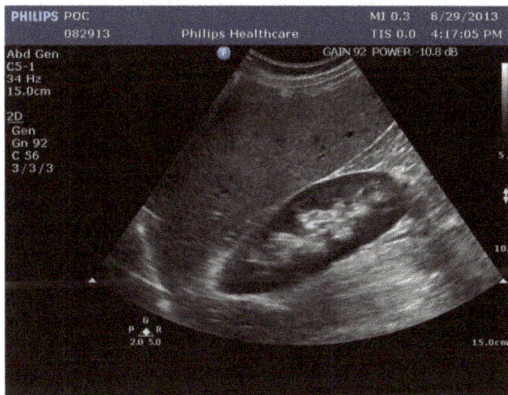

(B)

FIGURE 10-7. Image quality comparison at different power levels. (**A**) 0.0 dB or 100% power. (**B**) −10.8 dB, approximately 10% power.

Thermal index and mechanical index provide an indication of relative risk as operator controls are adjusted. The final benefit/risk assessment must include consideration of the index values and the medical needs of the patient. For each application, default settings that reflect current practice should be implemented.

No other imaging modality depends as strongly on operator ability. Misdiagnoses because of the opertor's lack of education, inexperience, or poor technique are more likely to cause harm than is the potential damage from ultrasound itself.

EDUCATIONAL USE

Medical professionals must be properly trained and this training must include scanning of human subjects. Scanning of human subjects for educational purposes should be supervised by trained professionals. Trainees should not attempt to scan themselves, a volunteer, or fellow trainee until proper instruction has been given. The instruction should include basic ultrasound physics and equipment controls. It should include the interaction of ultrasound energy with human tissue and the parameters used to measure and to limit that energy to acceptable levels under the output display standards. The trainee should also have a solid knowledge of the anatomy likely to be encountered within the part of the body to be scanned, so that the maximum educational benefit may be gained from the scanning session. The AIUM has provided guidelines regarding educational use involving human volunteers:

AIUM statement on Educational Use:

> When examinations are carried out for purposes of training or research, ultrasound exposures should be as low as reasonably achievable (ALARA) within the goals of the study/training. In addition, the subject should be informed of the anticipated exposure conditions and how these compare with normal diagnostic practice. Repetitive and prolonged exposures on a single subject should be justified and consistent with prudent and conservative use.

Scanning of pregnant volunteers for educational purposes requires special considerations. Recommendations by AIUM are summarized as follows. Subject participation should require appropriate informed content and the physician providing prenatal care should be informed of this participation. The pregnant individual should be afebrile and prescreened to attempt to avoid unexpected findings. A plan to address unexpected findings must be formulated. Scanning should not be performed in the first trimester. The teaching session should not exceed 1 hour per subject and pulsed Doppler mode is operated by the instructor only. The principle of ALARA is observed with limits of TI (≤ 1.0) and MI (< 1.9).

SUMMARY OF PATIENT SAFETY CONSIDERATIONS

- Diagnostic ultrasound has well-established medical applications with known benefits and recognized efficacy.

- No adverse biological effects related to the thermal mechanism have been demonstrated if the spatial peak, temporal average is less than 100 mW/cm^2 for unfocused beams and less than 1 W/cm^2 for focused beams or if the thermal index is less than 2.

- When nonthermal (mechanical) mechanism is considered, no adverse effects are associated with peak rarefactional pressures below 0.3 MPa or mechanical index less than 0.3.

- The obstetrical examination should be conducted with a thermal index less than 0.5, if possible. If the thermal index exceeds 2.5, the time should be limited to less than 1 minute and if the thermal index is 0.5 to 1, the time can be extended to 30 minutes. A mechanical index of less than 0.4 is recommended.

- For the non-obstetrical examination, a thermal index less than 2 may be used for scanning times on an extended basis. If the thermal index exceeds 6, then the time should be limited to less than 1 minute and if the thermal index is 2–6, then the time can be extended to 30 minutes. A mechanical index of less than 0.4 is recommended, but in the absence of gas bodies may be raised to as high as 1.9, if needed.

- Qualified health professionals with proper training and certification should conduct the examination at minimum power levels and scanning time to obtain the desired diagnostic information.

- The principle of ALARA, when applied, compels the operator to conduct the examination with the lowest reasonable exposure to the patient or subject. Exposure of the patient should be minimized by adjusting acquisition parameters whenever possible that contribute to energy deposition in the patient, while maintaining the desired information content.

- Thermal index and mechanical index provide an indication of relative risk as operator controls are adjusted. The final benefit/risk assessment must include consideration of the index values and the medical needs of the patient or educational benefit to be obtained in training or research.

- Scanning of human subjects as part of an educational program should be supervised by a trained ultrasound professional, and should only be attempted after specific educational requirements have been met.

- Ultrasonography during pregnancy should not be performed for the sole purpose of viewing the fetus by the mother or determining its sex or other "entertainment" use. Although the risk in these instances is very low, risk will always outweigh benefit where medical or educational benefit is absent.

References

American Institute of Ultrasound in Medicine: Medical ultrasound safety, ed 2, 2009.

Church CC, Carstensen EL, Nyborg WL, Carson PL, Frizzell LA, Bailey MR: The risk of exposure to diagnostic ultrasound in postnatal subjects: nonthermal mechanisms. J Ultrasound Med 27, 565–592, 2008.

Ewigman BG, Crane JP, Frigoletto FD, LeFevre ML, Bain RP, McNellis D: Effect of prenatal ultrasound screening on perinatal outcome. RADIUS Study Group, N Engl J Med 329, 821–827, 1993.

Hedrick WR: A Guide to Clinical Safety. Journal of Diagnostic Medical Sonography 21, 455–461, 2005.

Hedrick WR: Technology for diagnostic sonography, St. Louis, 2013, Elsevier.

Hedrick WR, Hykes DL: Biological Effects of Ultrasound Part I Specification of Intensity. Journal of Diagnostic Medical Sonography 7, 188–193, 1991.

Hedrick WR, Hykes DL: Biological Effects of Ultrasound Part II Interactions of Ultrasound with Matter. Journal of Diagnostic Medical Sonography 7, 194–196, 1991.

Hedrick WR, Hykes DL: Biological Effects of Ultrasound Part III In Vitro and Animal Studies. Journal of Diagnostic Medical Sonography 7, 264–269, 1991.

Hedrick WR, Hykes DL: Biological Effects of Ultrasound Part IV Epidemiologic Studies. Journal of Diagnostic Medical Sonography 7, 270–275, 1991.

Hedrick WR, Hykes DL: Biological Effects of Ultrasound Part V Clinical Safety. Journal of Diagnostic Medical Sonography 7, 333–338, 1991.

Hedrick WR, Hykes DL: An Overview of Thermal and Mechanical Output Indices. Journal of Diagnostic Medical Sonography 9, 228–235, 1993.

Hedrick WR, Hykes DL, Starchman DE: Ultrasound physics and instrumentation, ed 4, St. Louis, 2005, Elsevier.

Kremkau FW: Diagnostic ultrasound: principles and instruments, ed 8, Philadelphia, 2011, WB Saunders.

Miller MW, Nyborg WL, Dewey WC, Edwards MJ, Abramowicz JS, Brayman AA. Hyperthermic teratogenicity, thermal dose and diagnostic ultrasound during pregnancy: implications of new standards on tissue heating. Int J Hyperthermia 18, 361–384, 2002.

Nelson TR, Fowlkes JB, Abramowicz JS, et al: Ultrasound biosafety considerations for the practicing sonographer and sonologist. J Ultrasound Med 28, 139–150, 2009.

O'Brien Jr, Deng CX, Harris GR, et al: The risk of exposure to diagnostic ultrasound in postnatal subjects: thermal effects. J Ultrasound Med 27, 517–535, 2008.

Zagzebski JA: Essentials of ultrasound physics, St Louis, 1996, Mosby-Year Book.

Ziskin MC: The prudent use of diagnostic ultrasound. J Ultrasound Med 6, 415–416, 1987.

Index

Note: Page number followed by f and t indicates figure and table, respectively.

www.ingramcontent.com/pod-product-compliance
Lightning Source LLC
Chambersburg PA
CBHW081530220326
41598CB00036B/6386